The
D

HOW ONE WOMAN LET GO OF PERFECTION, FOUND HER CONFIDENCE, AND LOST OVER 220 POUNDS!

Judi Finneran

ISBN: 978-1-7366847-0-2 (Paperback)
Library of Congress Control Number: 2021912622

Front cover image by Tanja Prokop (www. bookcoverworld.com)
Book design by Andrea Reider (www. reiderbooks.com)
Book management by Liz Goodgold (www.RedFireBranding.com)

Printed and bound in the United States of America.

First printing edition 2021

JudiFinneran.com
748 South Meadows Parkway #A9-50
Reno, NV 89521
United States of America

www.JudiFinneran.com

FREE BONUS MATERIAL

Register Your Book Today and Get Valuable Bonus Material to Lose the Weight and Keep it Off!

I get it: losing weight is hard and keeping it off is even harder. I've assembled a host of goodies to help you with preparing, shopping, and tracking your food and goals. Just sign up here: www.TheBPlusDiet.com/bonus

Here's what you get for free just by signing up in one quick click:

1. **Food Tracker** – One of my core principles is "if you bite it, you write it." Folks who tracked every single bite lose twice as much weight as those who didn't.

2. **Gadget List** – After years of following my program, I've assembled a list of my favorite tools and gadgets to that help you in food prep.

3. **Weight Log** – Weighing yourself daily is key. This easy log lets you see your progress in action.

4. **100 Day Tennis Shoe Tracker** – Since I believe in visual reminders and accomplishments of goals, I've created a 100-day tracker. Set a goal and then color in every time you achieve that goal. Whether it's exercising daily, drinking your water, or avoiding alcohol, this is your way to see progress and results.

5. **Meal Planner** – Since planning your meal is the secret recipe for success, I recommend creating your meals one week at a time. This handy planner let's you see at a glance what you'll be eating, take notes and even keep a grocery list.

To your success, Judi

DEDICATION

This book is dedicated to my husband, Kevin, who has never judged me and has loved me through thick and thin – literally. And, to my four amazing children: Rachael, Michael, Dylan, and Patrick.

Acknowledgements

This book would never have become a reality without my wonderful book coach and sherpa, Liz Goodgold of RedFire Branding. Her guidance, suggestions, and support make it all possible. Thank you from the bottom of my heathy heart.

Introduction

I Lost the Weight and You Can Too!

It seems like forever, but I finally did it! And it was worth it! I have released the weight for good. Please don't misunderstand, I still follow the exact same program described in this book to stay at this weight. Every day I still focus on making the right choices. I can never eat the way I used to eat and weigh what I want to weigh and be happy with my weight. Change has to be permanent.

My journey is a wild ride. I was up, I was down. I was non-stop fighting with my weight for almost 50 years. I joined WW (formerly Weight Watchers) under at least 8 different names to avoid the embarrassment of having to admit I was back to take the weight off again.

Once I committed to this program and the weight started coming off, I had to share it with the world. I have many Facebook groups and coaching groups to help people just like you give up on the excuses and start a new way of living and eating.

"Judi is the best "Excuse Buster." If I gained or stalled, she always made me feel encouraged but at the same time

strongly encouraged accountability and transparency in analyzing if I had an excuse. Her coaching encouraged me to look within for those excuses and bring them into the light so I could move forward. These excuses were light bulb moments, and we often had a giggle over them especially when she would call herself an "excuse buster "because she had already thought of them all or made up herself. – Patrice

"*In December 2020, I signed on with Judi as my coach and began my weight loss journey. Thanks to Judi's steady, consistent, compassionate guidance, and support, I have lost 60 pounds so far and am well on my way to my personal goal weight. I am so grateful for her passion for sharing health and wellness with the world, and for her inspiring example that made me know I could do that, too.*" – Haley Steinhardt

Welcome to a Judgment-Free Zone

As you'll soon read, you can't tell me anything more embarrassing than the things I have done and suffered because of my weight. Yep, I actually ordered over 14 bags of onion rings from Jack in the Box and pretended they were for a party. They were just for me. Yes, I traveled with a seat belt extender because the regulation-size seat belt didn't fit around my girth. And, I admit to sitting on a chair only to watch it disintegrate under me.

I've bought "skinny" clothes and fat clothes – over and over again. Today, I only have one wardrobe. Whew! And everything in my closet fits today and will fit tomorrow.

"Judi is an inspiration. She is caring and absolutely non-judgmental. She shares her thoughts, her previous actions, and daily decisions that she makes on her journey to weight loss." - Bunni Lite

"This is the best book I have read about health and fitness. Judi has been my coach for years and now I feel I know her whole story. She has shared in an honest and down to earth way, a way that makes me feel motivated and inspired to continue on my own journey towards optimal health. I feel a connection to Judi's story, and I know you will as well." – Melissa Currier

Changing Your Mindset is Your Secret Weapon for Weight Loss

But, here's the secret. I only succeeded when I changed my mindset. I had to embrace the concept that I am in my weight loss battle for life. I had to say goodbye to "cheat" todays and embrace every day. Every day you either lose or you learn.

"Judi is my coach. My life is so much better because of being accountable to Judi. She has helped with reversing eating habits that have been out of control. She responds to me consistently and with positive comments about the progress I am making." - Myra Zuckerman

Once I realized that my mind and not my mouth controlled my weight, I was all in. I slowly converted to becoming a vegetarian and then a vegan. This program allows you to pick the vegetables you want; the protein you want. You don't have to eat a proscribed meal a la Jenny Craig or Nutrisystem. The B+ Diet is an abundance of veggies, protein, fruits, legumes, and flavor enhancers that you eat to fill you up with nourishment.

"Judi shares her experiences and has helped me through binge eating because she's been there. Judi is the best."
– Juanita T.

Food Is Fuel, You Don't Have to Be Perfect

But, here's the kicker. You don't have to be perfect. If you choose to have ice cream, you've chosen to have ice cream. You are not bad and ice cream is not evil; it's food! Afterall, having ice cream is not immoral, you will not gain all of the weight you lost because of one choice which does not support your weight loss goal. You make a choice and then go right back to your program. You don't give up, call it a "cheat day", and convince yourself that you might as well not even try. If you embrace this program as a way of life, you will succeed.

"Judi has been my coach for over 2 years. The most important lesson Judi taught me is that food is not the answer to feelings. Food is fuel. I started this way of life when grieving the loss of my first grandson. I had been using food to cope with emotions for years, and my weight had

steadily increased until I was considered obese. My health had declined, and I was at a crossroads. At the advice of my cardiologist, I started a whole food plant-based way of life, but I needed support. Just when I needed help most, I found Judi with her daily messages of encouragement.

I am down 90 pounds and maintain a normal BMI for 24 months now. When I start losing control, I go back to the basics and remember the lessons Judi taught me.

Judi Finneran saved my life." - Jeanie Schuldt

"Judi doesn't tell you what to do, she puts it on you. I love that about her. She truly cares. She knows that "I" am responsible for my choices." - Jerri Bozeman

"Losing and keeping weight off has always been a challenge for me. It wasn't until Judi invited me to join her on her journey that I began having success. Her encouragement, authenticity, and can-do attitude is an absolute inspiration. I'm excited and enthusiastic for the future and am confident because of Judi's support and coaching. She taught me that perfectionism is not my friend and when I embraced that, it was a game changer. She is amazing and when I count my blessings - I count her twice!" - Kathy Delapaz

If You Bite It, You Write It

In this program, you will track every morsel that goes in your mouth. You will weigh yourself every day. And, success is within reach.

> *"Writing down what I eat every single day have been what has helped keep me on track (literally! I track by hand every day!) I have lost over 70 lbs. since joining Judi in a Whole Food Plant-based lifestyle 2 1/2 years ago. Still a way to go, but I'm feeling more alive, more energetic, and loving life more as my natural weight is emerging."*
> – Mandy Kirk

> *"When I face a difficult situation or revert to my old unhealthy habits, rather than berate myself and give up entirely, I now ask myself, "What would Judi do?" She is a true role model."* – Linda Quezada

This Book is Your Life Changer

When you start following this program, you will feel better. You will have to work a little harder to ask for food that fits your needs; you may have to bring food with you so you make smarter choices; you may have to scope out restaurants before dining out, but you are firmly in control for life.

These are precious endorsements from folks who have worked with me on their own weight loss journey:

INTRODUCTION

"Great book full of tips and strategies for achieving and maintaining long-term weight loss. The B+ Diet isn't just another diet; it can change your life!" - Kristen Scott

"The B+ Diet gave me permission to stop dieting and focus on a permanent lifestyle change instead." - Karine Tovmassian

"Finally, a book that tells the truth about weight loss! Through her book, The B+ Diet, Judi becomes the coach that everyone who's ever struggled with weight loss has been waiting for. She's a leader that knows the way and shows the way to become healthy, happy, and free from ever dieting again." -Milan Jensen

"Judi Finneran has been invaluable to me in my weight loss journey. Her knowledge, daily good habits and modeling behaviors are incomparable! Her empathy and patience are exceptional! She can help ANYONE lose weight and gain health if they really want it." - Traci Jones

"Judi has inspired me; I'm learning from my setbacks and she never makes me feel belittled." – Dianna V

"A genuinely warm and caring person, Judi coaches from the heart. She knows and selflessly shares what it takes to succeed. Her advice is pure magic!" - Chris

"What an inspiration for me at 84 years old: plant-based meals, low in calories, high in nutrients, and no more yoyo diets – and following Judi's journey. She coaches and encourages many of us daily." - Char DuBay

"If you ever suffered from the pain and humiliation of being overweight, Judi will show you that no matter how long or how deeply you have suffered there is hope. With Judi's guidance and a few simple healthy hacks, like drinking more water and eating more vegetables, you too can achieve the health and the body that you so richly deserve". - Chef AJ, author of the bestselling *The Secrets to Ultimate Weight Loss*

I am here for you. Connect with me for how I can support you on your journey.

Judi@JudiFinneran.com
Facebook: https://www.facebook.com/JudiAFinneran
Website: https://thebplusdiet.com/
Instagram: https://www.instagram.com/judifinneran/
2B Mindset: https://tinyurl.com/2bveganmindset

Table of Contents

Part I: The Weight-Loss Journey

Part II: The Whole Enchilada—
The Entire B+ Program

CHAPTER 1

The Winning Recipe

Changing Your Lifestyle to Change Your Weight

"My weaknesses have always been food and men—in that order." —Dolly Parton

D iets do work. If followed, each results in weight loss. I speak from personal experience: I have tried at least 80 percent of the diets out there and lost weight every time. We often hear that "diets don't work"; I don't believe it for a minute. My experience has been that when you are "on a diet," you change the way you eat, the food you eat, and the amount you eat for a set time frame. While "doing the diet," you lose weight if you are following the plan as prescribed.

All Diets Work

When we reach our goal weight or quit the diet, most of us revert to the way we ate before starting the diet. Sometimes slowly or sometimes quickly, the weight we lost comes back. The problem with diets is that the focus is on losing weight instead of making permanent lifestyle changes.

Here is a list of some of the diets I have tried, and all of them worked in the short term:

- Atkins
- Medifast
- Lindora
- Jenny Craig
- Nutrisystem
- Optifast
- Food Combining (Fit for Life)
- Weight Watchers

I was remarkably successful on all of these diets. For example, my first time on Nutrisystem, I lost 79 pounds. On Lindora, I lost 65+ pounds the first time. On Jenny Craig, I lost over 70 pounds the first time. Optifast resulted in 150 pounds lost in ten months, the first time. Are you noticing a trend here?

My biggest weight loss and success on each diet was during the *first* time on each of them.

The kicker is that on each of these diets I regained (or found) every pound I lost, and each pound brought a few new friends with them. I was a fabulous dieter. I am coachable and I can follow instructions, almost obsessively, and so I lost weight.

Becoming the Queen of the Lost-and-Found Department

At one point, I decided to try and figure out how much weight I had lost and found. And to my horror and amazement, I had lost and found over 2,500 pounds since I became an adult! I'm pretty sure 2,200 pounds is the weight of a large bison or a Volkswagen. This is when I realized I had become the Queen of the Weight Lost-and-Found Department—a crown I was not proud to accept.

How had this happened to me? I believe I am an intelligent woman, and yet how had I become so dumb as to let this lose-gain cycle continue? This book is my story of finding my confidence, letting go of becoming perfect, and finally losing the weight.

Why Shaming Shapes Us Forever

When I look back at photos of me as a kid, I see that I began to look a little chubby about third or fourth grade. Previously, I didn't have a weight problem or an image issue.

The first time I remember being embarrassed by my weight was as a high school freshman. It was the first day of school in my PE class and everyone was getting weighed in on a balance beam scale by the gym teacher. We stood in a long line awaiting our turn to weigh in as the teacher's assistant recorded the number. The assistant was at the end of the line, so the teacher had to shout out the weight of each girl as we stood on the scale. Seriously, what was that about? I was nervous and dreading stepping up on that scale and having everyone hear what I weighed. On top of that, we were in a school gymnasium in which sound carried, and there were other groups of people in the gymnasium. I can remember even now what I was wearing—a blue-and-white sailor suit type skirt and top. When it was my turn, she moved the little weight along the bar until it stopped and she shouted at the back of the line, "165 pounds." I was 5 feet, 4 inches tall, and this meant I was overweight.

I had never been on a diet, thought about a diet, or as far as I can remember, thought about what I weighed up until that moment in my life. I just knew I was embarrassed and felt bad about myself.

When I was a sophomore in high school, my mom started going to TOPS (Take Off Pounds Sensibly), a weekly meeting where each member would get weighed in. Get this: if you gained weight, you had to sit in the Pig Pen! I don't recall if my mom lost weight. I do remember that she went with a group of other ladies, who all got ice cream to celebrate afterwards, knowing they had another week before they had to "weigh in" again. I see the beginning of my pattern of losing, gaining, and "cheating" starting here.

When my mom was on TOPS, I decided to lose weight too and somehow must have heard about the Atkins Diet. All I remember is broiling lots of hamburger patties with slices of cheddar cheese on top and eating lots of cottage cheese. It worked and I got down to 130 pounds, which was a good weight for me. I maintained this weight throughout the rest of high school and into college.

My goal at the time was to become an airline stewardess (they were not called flight attendants back then), and I knew I had to hit a certain weight. I wanted to fly for Pan Am, the prestigious airline of the day. I planned on learning French, because you had to speak at least one foreign language. Becoming a stewardess was going to allow me to travel the world, which was a dream of mine then and still is. And, when I became too old to work as a stewardess, my plan was to take my language skills and work at the United Nations. I had big goals.

From tenth grade through my first year of college, I had one boyfriend, and when we broke up, I was devastated. I met someone new and the relationship progressed very quickly— the next thing I knew I was engaged and getting married when I was just 20½ years old. Something inside of me knew this was a rebound relationship and was a big mistake.

The night before the wedding, my fiancé dropped me off at Mom's house, where my mom and my future mother-in-law were cutting up pineapple in the kitchen for the reception the next day. I still can visualize where everyone was standing when I said, "This is a mistake and I am not ready to get married."

5

They both looked at me horrified and then chuckled. They reassured me that my feelings were simply pre-wedding jitters and perfectly normal. Even though I knew they were wrong, I didn't have the courage to challenge them. Here I was at 20 years old, with 400 people coming to a Catholic church the next morning, seven attendants with dresses made by my grandmother, and I didn't want to get married. But I swallowed my indecision, woke up the next morning, and got married.

Bite-Sized Nugget

Listen to your gut ... and your stomach. Sometimes you're not hungry but are using food to reward or punish yourself.

The Beginning of Bingeing: When You Start Hiding Your Food, You're in Trouble!

Without realizing it, I quickly gained 25 pounds while I was engaged. Clearly, it was because I was engaged to someone I really didn't want to marry. However, I had no reference for that kind of thinking then.

It never dawned on me I was eating because I was unhappy and "stuffing my feelings down" with food. I remember the first time I used food to punish myself and anesthetize myself from my feelings. It was a Monday morning, June 21. I had been married two days prior and had just spent the first night in my new apartment with my new husband. When he left for work,

I sat there alone, never allowing myself to ask even consciously "What have I done?" Instead, I was lonely and feeling as though I had just sealed my fate by giving up on my dreams.

Next door to our apartment building was a convenience store. I walked on over and bought a box of doughnuts (the eight-piece variety box). I ate every single one of them. When I was done, I threw the box away in the large garbage containers for the apartment building. I was too embarrassed to put the box in our trash where it would be evidence of what I had just done—my first binge-eating experience. It might have been the first, but it certainly wouldn't be the last.

Bite-Sized Nugget
Shame doesn't belong in any diet.

I never mentioned this episode to anyone because I must have been ashamed without even knowing why. Instinctively, I realized that eating a box of doughnuts, keeping it a secret, and hiding the evidence was not the right thing for me to do. The first step on the road to becoming the Queen of the Weight Lost-and-Found Department had been taken. The battle with losing and finding weight had begun and would continue for the next forty years.

Over the first six months of my marriage, I managed to put on a whopping 50 pounds. When people looked at me funny, I blamed it on birth control pills, and people pretended to believe me. Seriously, birth control pills? I had never learned how to cook, so Hamburger Helper and Kraft Macaroni and Cheese became staples in our house. It didn't help that we went out to dinner with my parents at least once a week, and Sunday dinners at my in-laws were always big Italian meals.

I had traded my dreams and goals for a husband who wasn't the right one for me and a bunch of boxed meals and unhappiness.

IN A NUTSHELL

1. All diets work; it's your plan on how to change your eating habits forever that determines your success.
2. It's true: shift your mindset and you shift the results.

CHAPTER 2

Sneak and Eat

Why Binge Eating Is the First Danger Sign

"There are only two mistakes one can make along the road to truth; not going all the way and not starting." —Buddha

My weight continued to climb in the early years of my first marriage and I did little about it. When I got married, I was a server at a restaurant across the street from Disneyland and we had to wear these ugly uniforms. They were a goldish-tan color dress with buttons up the front and straight up and down. When we put our aprons on, it made a waist, sort of. I'd been married a couple of months when my manager called me over and told me my uniform was too tight and I needed to trade it in for the next size up. Mortifying, to say the least! I had reached the fantasy point in my mind when you believe no one else has noticed all the weight you have gained.

Bite-Sized Nugget
The first step in making a change is realizing you need to change.

My marriage was crumbling little bits at a time. Although my husband worked full-time, he also had a passion for singing. He joined a band, and the group actually got gigs! At first, the wives of the band members would attend the act, but being an audience member so many times over got old. To put it in perspective, my hubby would leave around 5 p.m. every night and not be home until at least 2 a.m. That left a lot of hours for a newlywed bride to be sitting at home wondering what her husband was doing. I soon realized food could be a good distraction.

This time period is when my binge eating bloomed, and like most bad habits, it began slowly and quickly escalated. Kraft Macaroni and Cheese became a close friend, with me devouring an entire box right after he left. At that time, you could get five boxes on sale for $1.00, and I stocked up on them. I felt guilty eating that quantity of food; I knew it wasn't normal or healthy.

Then the next time he traveled, I made two boxes and ate the whole thing. Eventually, my mac 'n' cheese habit reached a high of three boxes per sitting. But in public around other people, I would eat normally.

The Beginning of Sneak and Eat: My Dangerous Downfall

Sometime later we moved into a new apartment, and the two most vivid memories I have of this apartment are of onion rings and hiding in the shower. Our new place was right down the street from a Jack in the Box, and I really liked their onion rings. So, one Friday night when I was alone, I went through the drive-through and bought two orders of onion rings. I discovered the appeal and allure of drive-throughs for sneak eating and how wonderful it was not to have to get out of your car. By the time I got home, one order would be almost gone, and the other quickly followed. Even I was too embarrassed to go back again, so I waited until the next night and got three orders of onion rings. Our apartment was upstairs. No matter what the weather was, I would open the windows in the den where I ate while watching TV so the smell of the onion rings would not fill the room. As soon as I was done, I would take all the trash out to the dumpsters, brush my teeth, and scrub my hands.

Being in that den with the door closed and the television on was like being in my own little world. A cave where I felt safe and did not have to think about why my husband was getting home at 3:00 a.m. or 3:30 a.m. instead of 2:00 a.m. He would say the guys all went out to breakfast, and maybe they did, but who knew? Not me. As the number of orders increased, I even started getting embarrassed to go to the drive-through, but not enough to stop doing it. When the number of orders got to nine (I vowed to never get to double digits, and yet I peaked at thirteen orders), I told the fast-food workers they need not put each order in individual bags, but simply combine them. Picture my embarrassment when I drove up to pay and the girl asked me what I was doing with all these onion rings. I quickly answered that we had a poker game going on at my house and I was sent out for snacks. That was the last time I went there.

One night I had eaten so many onion rings, I felt sick to my stomach and had a pounding headache. I told myself I had eaten so much that the food was backed up to my head. My lips and insides felt coated with grease, and I was also sick at heart. When my husband got home, around 2:00 a.m. for a change, he brought me a treat. Yes, he brought me a bag of onion rings from Jack in the Box! As I looked at them, I imagined this was my punishment or karma for being such a horrible person. Of course, I had to eat them or he would wonder what was wrong.

The apartments we lived in had covered parking spots instead of garages, so it was easy to see if people we knew were home or not. One night, I was in the den bingeing on onion rings, when someone knocked at the door. I could not imagine who it was and ignored it. The knocking got louder and I heard someone calling my name, and I realized it was a neighbor I knew. I was so horrified to be found hoarding onion rings that I hid in my own bathroom shower until she went away. As I stood there, I realized I was sick, and I did not want to live like this any longer.

Bite-Sized Nugget

Your desire to change must be greater than your desire to stay the same.

The next day, I found out where there was a Weight Watchers meeting near me. Within a week, I joined my very first Weight Watchers meeting. While Weight Watchers was not going to be the final answer for me, it worked for a while and I started learning a few new habits.

IN A NUTSHELL

1. Recognize the symptoms of bingeing. It's not healthy to overeat, order copious amounts of food, or hide the evidence.
2. Ensure you're clear that you're not swallowing your feelings. Eating because you're lonely or unhappy will only make you more miserable.

CHAPTER 3

Carrot and Stick

The Merry-Go-Round of Losing and Gaining

"We cannot start over, but we can begin again and make a new ending."—Zig Ziglar

When I went to my first Weight Watchers meeting, I was terrified to walk in the door and mortified I had to be there. I was getting used to worrying I would be the heaviest person there. Even worse was stepping up on that scale; it was the balance beam kind, just like the one in my freshman year in high school. However, instead of the non-chalant (and insensitive) gym teacher shouting out my weight to someone at the end of the line with a clipboard, there was a very nice woman named Rhoda who smiled nicely and wrote my weight into a little white booklet and closed it very quickly. I really wish I had kept my first Weight Watchers book so I would know exactly what I weighed that day. I am guessing my weight was between 180 and 190 pounds, which put me at least 60 pounds over my ideal weight. It seemed impossible to me at that time to lose 60 pounds, not knowing years later I would be excited when I "only" had 60 pounds more to lose.

Welcome to Weight Watchers: Watching It Come Off ... and On

This was back in the days of the "original" Weight Watchers program, the one created by Jean Nidetch. It was nothing like the plan today where you can have anything you want, as long as you count the points. Jean Nidetch created this plan from a diet booklet she was given by the City or County of New York. The plan detailed exactly what you were to eat each day and each week:

- No more than four eggs per week
- Eat fish five times a week (canned tuna and I become new BFFs)
- Eat liver once a week (the only guideline I did not faithfully follow every week)
- Three fruits daily, and only one could be an apple or a banana
- Four ounces of protein at lunch and six ounces of protein at dinner

- Unlimited #3 vegetables (non-starchy)
- One serving daily of #4 vegetables (starchy)

I am sure there were guidelines about bread and other things. And there was a very specific list of what not to eat at the back of the food program guide. We were given a food diary to record everything we ate; three squares down for each meal and seven columns across for the days of the week. Along the bottom were the boxes for the weekly choices. Eggs followed by four little boxes, fish followed by five little boxes, and the one dreaded box for liver.

By this time, I was working for Orange County in the tax assessor's office. My friend and I had found a little lounge across the street from our office in a bank building, and that is where we ate lunch every day. I wished I had known about Weight Watchers a couple of years earlier. In my first year of marriage, I had a job which I really liked, working at Orange County Medical Center. At the time I was hired, I was as least 50 pounds overweight, and employment laws were much different then. I had a pre-employment physical and was told I had to lose those 50 pounds within six months to keep my job. Imagine that happening now. I was not losing any weight, and as the end of those six months came closer, I gave up and just quit my job. I had to leave a job because I was too heavy.

Being the compliant, coachable Weight Watchers member and good rule-follower, I was committed to following the plan exactly. When a few weeks into the program I learned I was messing up by having two eggs for breakfast (only one was allowed on each of four days), I felt guilty I had done it wrong. Budding perfectionist showing up!

Bite-Sized Nugget
Persistence, not perfection.

I reached my goal weight in seven months and had never gone off plan, with the exception of the egg misunderstanding (oh, and the liver, which I could only handle two or three times). Upon achieving your goal weight, you were moved to an eight-week maintenance plan, where all the foods you had not been allowed to eat were transitioned back into your diet. Each week you got a new little insert booklet for your food program, adding all of the previously forbidden foods back. The idea was to gradually reintroduce these foods into your diet.

As I had done in the previous months, I followed the plan to the letter—until week eight, the last week in the maintenance program. This final week of maintenance was when you got to choose a meal of anything you wanted once a month. Well, this was music to my ears, and I chose my favorite food of all, Mexican food. My husband and I went out to dinner. Almost everything I ordered were things I had not had for months, and like in the old onion ring days, I ate and ate and ate until I was almost sick. Eight months of tracking, following the plan, and in one night it seemed it all went out the window. I am not really sure what happened that night other than that I started gaining the weight back again.

At some point, the weight gain was not okay, and I decided to return to Weight Watchers and "start over." Famous last words: start over. Not restart, not get back onto the program, but start over. Because I had reached my weight-loss goal and completed maintenance, I was a "Lifetime Member," which meant I could go back at any time and not have to pay a fee to rejoin. All I would be required to do was to pay the weekly fee until I was back to within two pounds of my goal weight.

However, admitting I had gained my weight back felt like admitting being a failure. When rejoining I did not tell them I'd been a member before; I simply paid the fee to join, got a new little white booklet, and started over. It also meant I could not go back to the meeting I had attended previously, since people would know me there. So, I found a different meeting.

After attending a couple of weeks and not following the program, I quit again. And then a few weeks or months later I would join another new meeting, and then another and another. At the time I was living in Orange County, so there were a lot of meetings to choose from. And each time I found a new meeting to join, I would have gained a few more pounds. Luckily or not, this was before everything was computerized, and if a member did not attend meetings for a number of weeks, their card was purged from the system and there was no easy way at the local meeting to track who had and had not been a member before.

The Elusive Goal of Hitting Goal Weight

This went on for probably a year until I found a meeting which stuck, and I was able to reach my goal weight and become a Lifetime Member again. Still, I started gaining the weight back and the whole cycle would begin again. This was certainly not serving me in any way, and each time I rejoined as a new member, I was affirming to myself that I would never be able to achieve and maintain my goal weight and I was a failure and a quitter. I established a pattern which would go on for years—joining, quitting, and starting over. At some point, I worried someone would find out what I was doing and wonder why I was joining and starting over at so many different meetings and paying the join-up fee every time. My answer to this was to make up names, and as long as I paid cash, no one knew the difference. Yes, I joined under made-up names.

Starting My Career as a
Weight-Loss Leader

My marriage ended seven years after it had begun. Most of those years I spent losing and finding weight. About nine months before we separated, I joined a meeting at the Orange Mall with my next-door neighbor. This was the first time I had done this with a friend, a support person, and I believe it really made a difference. After having joined twenty to twenty-five times, reaching Lifetime Member status at least five times, this time I joined with my real name, continued to my goal weight, and became a Lifetime Member for the last time. The months leading up to reaching my goal weight, I was invited to assist the group leader with the meeting by helping to weigh in people at the meeting. I really liked and admired Pat, my group leader, and she was a big influence on my success. My weight mostly stabilized while I continued through my divorce, a bad relationship, and changing jobs.

When I got engaged to Kevin, I went back to this same meeting (huge progress for me) to lose just a bit of weight before I got married. I was so happy Pat was still there. In fact, Pat attended my wedding. During this time, I decided I wanted to be a group leader. (This was the first step to my becoming a Healthy Weight Coach many years later.) I remembered how much I had loved weighing people in and talking with them and encouraging them. Supporting them helped me stay motivated. Pat was totally supportive of my idea and very encouraging, and I started the training to become a leader. Pat's class at the Orange Mall was one of the biggest in the county. It was consistently attended by fifty to sixty members and often grew to over a hundred or more in January each year.

I loved my training and was excited with the idea of sharing my story, my ideas, and my suggestions with members on how to reach their goal weights and stay there. When the training was finished, you were assigned a class of your very own.

Imagine my surprise when I was asked to take over Pat's classes at the Orange Mall. Pat was offered a job with the corporate offices and I took over all three of her classes in Orange. All were on Tuesday: one at 2:00 p.m., another at 4:00 p.m., and "my class" at 6:00 p.m. It was pretty scary going from sitting in the front row, always my seat of choice, to standing in the front of the room. I was shocked when I was asked to become the leader of the class I had been attending for so long and sad that Pat was not going to be my leader any longer. This was a huge honor and vote of confidence and (did I mention) very scary.

Like me, all of the other members loved Pat and were extremely disappointed she would be gone. Also, Pat did not get an opportunity to say goodbye. If we as leaders were going to be gone on vacation or miss a meeting for any reason, we did not tell the class ahead of time. There was a concern that if the members knew their leader was not going to be there, they might skip the meeting. I took over the classes and loved them. Since I was working in Anaheim and lived in Carlsbad, I stated picking up some more classes along the I-5 on my way home, and pretty soon, I had classes five days a week.

Sadly, this past year Pat passed away without me being able to tell her once more how much her faith in me meant and how it would so deeply impact the work I do today.

As leaders, we attended monthly training and staff meetings where we had to weigh in. To keep our classes, we had to stay within two pounds of our goal, and this was great motivation to stay on track.

Pregnancy and Weight Gain

I did this for two years until I found a new job in San Diego. I had to give up several of my classes in Orange County and added a few in San Diego. Then I got pregnant. I had maintained a steady weight for three years, the longest stretch for me since I was 20. During my first pregnancy, I had all-day sickness as opposed to morning sickness and was not gaining any weight. At one of my early OB appointments, my doctor was worried about this and told me I needed to gain some weight. Seriously? No one had ever told me that before, and being the coachable person I am, I gained sixty pounds by the time my daughter was born.

When Rachael was twelve weeks old, she became sick. Over the next couple of months with many scares and hospitalizations we learned she had a very rare neurological disorder called Aicardi syndrome, named after the French pediatrician who discovered it. I was standing by my Rachael's bed alone (Kevin had gone to the cafeteria or something) in the hospital when her pediatric neurologist walked into the room and said, "Your daughter has Aicardi syndrome, which means she is profoundly handicapped, and it can lead to early death."

Then he walked out of the room. Bam, talk about a sucky bedside manner. Aicardi syndrome is a rare genetic disorder characterized by the partial or complete absence of a key structure in the brain called the corpus callosum, the presence of retinal abnormalities, and seizures in the form of infantile spasms. It only occurs in girls. At this time, Rachael was one of only about two hundred diagnosed cases in the world. In the hospital over the next few months, Rachael would often have up to eighty seizures a day. I can't even remember how many different anti-convulsants she was on. Some medicines helped in the short term, and except for a few months when she was seizure-free, she continues to have them. Rachael is 100 percent dependent on care and can't talk, walk, or sit up, etc. However, she has the most amazing smile you can imagine. She lived at home with us until she was 22. She now lives in a great group home close to us.

Twenty months later Michael was born. Three years later Patrick and Dylan, my twins, were born. Once again, I had some weight to lose. I had literally just reached my goal weight again when I found I was pregnant with twins. In fact, on Christmas Eve at my mom's house, one of the gifts I opened from her was some lovely, sexy lingerie. She laughed and said, "Now just don't get pregnant again." Kevin and I looked at each other and smiled, and that is when I told my parents I was not only pregnant, but I was also having twins.

Bite-Sized Nugget

Stop the failure mentality. If you chose to splurge, it's OK – just get back on track the next day. We only run into trouble when a splurge causes us to stop our life-long commitment to stay at a healthy weight.

IN A NUTSHELL

1. One setback is just a setback; you are human and you're not perfect. You don't have to start over. Just keep moving ahead and keep your eyes on the goal.
2. Take a risk. All of life is a risk, and you decide what makes sense for you.

CHAPTER 4

Chewing the Fat

Emotional Eating and Its Weapons of Mass Consumption

"Don't reward yourself with food. You are not a dog."
—Anonymous

Welcome to our tumultuous year of 1990. We were 18 months into our five-year plan to relocate from sunny California to Maui, Hawaii. Having visited there for a family vacation, we knew this place was paradise. We believed that with a strategic plan, we could get there. After all, Kevin just needed a job, I needed to plan my new career in real estate, we had to sell our house in San Diego, enroll children in school (including two who were only six months old plus our special needs daughter), and corral everyone, including the dog, to an island home almost three thousand miles away.

Aloha, Hawaii!

You know what they say about plans. One year into our plan, my husband was offered a job transfer opportunity in Maui. You have to understand that Kevin worked for Kaiser Permanente, and each facility only had one biomed tech. These jobs virtually never materialize. And yet here it was, right within our grasp. We both took ahold of the chance of a lifetime to move to Hawaii.

Kevin needed to be there almost immediately, so he went ahead of me and the kids by about six months. I stayed in California working full-time, raising four children (all in diapers), one dog, and dealing with the details of moving across an ocean. I initially tried selling our house, but the California real estate market had collapsed. Our house was now worth 75 percent less than what we paid for it. We had no alternative but to rent out our brand-new San Diego home while simultaneously looking for a place to rent in Hawaii. As I organized, packed, and shipped everything, the four children and I moved into my mom's house for the last thirty long days before joining Kevin.

Losing the Comfort of
My Safety Net and Blanket

Everyone's relationship with their mom is complicated. I knew my mom didn't want me to move so far away, especially since my dad had recently passed. I understood her feelings. She also thought I was crazy for leaving my "dream job." Yep, I too was employed at Kaiser, but as a customer relations manager devoted to recruiting and retaining big clients. As a result, I had a company car, unlimited expense account, season tickets to the Padres, Chargers, symphony, etc. I was quitting my job, giving up all of these perks, and would start a new career in Hawaii. Scary!

As I figuratively talked myself off the limb of the fear tree, I started to ask myself, "What's the worst that can happen?" I'd always dreamed that living in Hawaii would be like winning the sunny lottery. But if need be, the entire family would move back to San Diego.

Bite-Sized Nugget

Ask yourself, "What's the worst that can happen?" What you're doing isn't working, so you might as well try something new and jump!

Here's the interesting thing: during those six months without Kevin in which I was overworked and overwhelmed, I lost almost 70 pounds! It wasn't by accident, but by intention using Nutrisystem. As is clear throughout this book, all diets work. You just must choose a mindset and an eating plan that you can stay on for life.

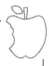

You can't spell challenge without change. I was focused on studying for my new real estate career, taking care of infant twins plus two other children, juggling strollers and a wheelchair, and yet I was committed to surprising my husband with a massive weight loss when I stepped off that plane in Hawaii. And I did. The look on his face was priceless.

Most people would have thought that I had valid excuses for gaining weight during that period. As I now repeat constantly to my clients: there are no excuses. You *choose* what you put in your mouth. You had a choice and made choices which caused the weight gain.

Facing the Reality of Real Estate

I passed my Hawaii real estate exam, which was the essential first step in launching my new career in Maui. In essence, I was leaving a salaried job for a commission-only arrangement. I partnered with Cara, a brilliant agent on the island. With her by my side, I earned a PhD in real estate, although very little money.

I remember the day I turned down a listing because the seller wanted more money than was realistic. It was the right decision because it saved time, energy, and any feelings of ill-will. As Cara reinforced, you've haven't earned your stripes as a realtor until you've turned down your first big listing. The issue, of course, was that I turned down the listing without having a book of business. After nine months of being in real estate, my commission remained a big, fat zero.

I knew I had core principles which applied regardless of what business I'm in. Today, they remain as follows:

- **Integrity:** Never sell your soul; do what's right.
- **Honesty:** I'm honest to a fault.
- **Realism:** I don't believe in fantasy worlds; whether it takes six months to sell a house or nine months to lose the weight, I always provide a realistic perspective.
- **Strong work ethic:** I never quit because the work is too hard. Do the work and the results will follow.

Bite-Sized Nugget

When people are gaining weight, they lose track of time. When they are trying to lose weight, they lose perspective. Weight loss takes longer than you think it will.

Our biggest issue in Hawaii was the schools. Three days a week, Michael attended an amazing preschool that we loved and that he enjoyed. Just as she had been in California, Rachael was in special education; however, the services offered at that time were not on par with what we were used to in California. We worried she was not being given the opportunity to maximize her potential.

The Guilt and Failure Complex

The killer combination of poor schools and no commissions finally convinced us that we had to move back to San Diego. I felt as if I were heading home with my tail between my legs and as an utter failure. I also had vague visions of my mother uttering: "I told you so."

Once again, Kevin and I would be separated by 2,537 miles. I moved back to California and my mom allowed us to stay with her until the tenants moved out of our house and Kevin returned. Yes, the kids, dog, and I moved back, and Kevin had to stay on Maui until he found a job in California. Finding a job in California while living in Hawaii was extremely difficult. Kevin was not able to move back for one full year!!!!

While my mom was very gracious to let us stay with her while waiting for Kevin to get a job and join us in back in California, there was also a ton of stress. Feeling like a failure in not making Hawaii work, not having any income while having to kick off my real estate business and missing my husband all led me right back to emotional eating again. I basically ate all of my feelings.

I felt that since my life was so crazy, why even try to maintain the weight? Heck, I could gain weight faster than anyone! Just watch me! And watch me they did. I ballooned in weight quite quickly.

At the same time that Kevin was working to find a job in California, I was ready to apply my newly honed real estate skills in a market that I knew quite well. I interviewed with many real estate offices and chose one I really liked. I applied my strong work ethic. In my first year, I sold twelve houses, which was significantly better than my results in Hawaii. Still, the stress of missing Kevin, acting as a single mom of four, and dealing with feelings of failure led me down a horrific path of overeating.

IN A NUTSHELL

1. Staying on a lifetime plan of wellness takes work, especially during times of stress. Whether you're moving, dealing with kids, staying with your mom, or working, you must plan "me" time to stay focused.
2. Stop eating your feelings. It won't make you feel any better and you'll end up heavier than where you are now.

CHAPTER 5

Menu for Success

Why Coaching Always Belongs on Your Plate!

"If you want something different, do something different."
—Anonymous

In my first year of being a realtor back in California, I learned about the Mike Ferry Organization and started attending some of its training events. I very much enjoyed the way Mike taught and agreed with his style and became what we called a "Ferryite." I made a point to attend as many trainings as possible and put his systems to work, which they did! I learned better presentation skills, how to handle objections, and how to track my numbers. When their program offered the opportunity to have someone coach me, I signed up right away. The coaching call was a 15- to 20-minute call every two weeks with a coach who worked for the Mike Ferry Organization. While I was not that impressed with my first coach, I liked the idea of accountability and having someone know what I said I was going to do and me reporting back that I did it. It was a great experience to learn to be accountable to someone else.

Mike held an annual event called the Superstar Retreat each August in Palm Desert, California, and I signed up to go. There were more than 1,000 people there my first year. People, many of them in their pajamas or workout clothes, slept outside the door to get the best spots. I actually did get in line around 3 a.m., fully dressed for the event by the way, and ended up in an end row seat about twenty rows back. I was glued to everything Mike shared and how clearly he made success seem like a system in which "if you follow the steps, you will achieve success." I believed it then and I still believe it today, even more strongly. I felt I was meant to be there when Mike was sharing something, and then HE looked directly at me and referred to me as the lady wearing white in an example.

The Power of Goal Setting and Affirmations

One of the topics Mike talked about was the power of affirmations and how focusing on what is important to us and setting goals and believing in them helps us to achieve those goals. When I got back to my office, I invited a couple of other people to do the Mike Ferry system with me, and we would support each other. At home, I started getting up earlier and created a morning routine. On the first morning, I made a list of twenty affirmations, several of which had to do with weight loss, healthy weight, what size clothes I wore, etc. And for months I repeated them out loud, rewrote, tweaked, and focused on these same twenty affirmations. For whatever reason, a few months down the line, I stopped doing them. Whether you call them goals or affirmations, there is power in knowing where you want to go and how to get there.

The next year, three of my friends from my office joined me at the Superstar Retreat. A couple of major things happened at this second event. One was that Mike shared that he had spent the last year personally one-on-one coaching twelve realtors on a weekly basis. With the coaching, these realtors' businesses had exploded. They shared on a panel how the heightened account-ability of coaching with Mike inspired them to do more, be better, and push harder in their business; as a result, they exceeded their own expectations. Mike said he was going to do one-on-one coaching again with another twelve people. A good friend of his and great realtor, Tim, was going to coach this group with him. This was his launch of the Mike Ferry One-on-One Coaching Program. Nervous and excited, my friend Susan and I filled out the applications. Only twenty-four people were going to be chosen, and the cost was $1,000 a month. Yikes. So, we just had to wait and see.

Although I did not recognize it as such at the time, the next major thing that affected my professional development was a speaker Mike had invited to present to us at the end of the day. Attendance was optional. Mike had become involved with a company that sold health products, and the guest speaker was there to share information on health. The presenter, Inger, was a nutritionist and health coach.

Her presentation was the first time I heard some new terms, such as "free radicals." She mentioned a book called *Fit for Life* by Marilyn and Harvey Diamond. I remembered it because years before my sister-in-law was using their food combining theory to lose weight. When I got home, I purchased the book and read it. Two things happened.

First, I decided to try food combining, and I began losing weight. I think the weight loss didn't actually come from food combining but from being aware of what I was eating and focusing on eating only healthy food.

One Commitment at a Time: Why I Gave Up Chicken

Second, the book discussed the processing of chicken for food. I was turned off and decided I was not going to eat poultry any longer. When I told Kevin, he was fine with that and said he never really liked chicken all that much anyway. Without knowing it, that was my first step toward becoming vegetarian and then vegan. It all began with making just one commitment.

Bite-Sized Nugget

Coaching works because the fees and partnership hold you accountable to yourself! It just might be the secret weapon you need to achieve your goals.

A few weeks after the event, I got "the call" that I had been accepted into the One-on-One Coaching Program and that Tim was going to be my coach. This included a 30-minute call every week, which cost me $250 dollars per call—so I intended to do everything he said. When I did the coaching program the first time, I was not as vested, but this time I was totally committed. If I was going to be paying that much money to someone to tell me what to do, I was going to listen to him and do it! Plus, he was selling real estate NOW and doing daily the same things he was suggesting I do. That was the difference. The other coaches weren't selling real estate and did not have the same credibility with me.

The Accountability Factor

Many of us resist having someone hold us accountable. When we share our plans or goals with others, we are allowing ourselves to be vulnerable. When we keep our goals secret, it is much easier to rationalize away why we did not follow through. People tell me frequently they don't set goals because they failed in the past and they don't want to be disappointed again. Or they say if they tell someone what they are doing, they will have to actually do it. We have all set goals we did not meet, and what is important is what we learned from that experience. Sometimes even when we don't reach the goals we set, we may have accomplished a lot more than if we had not been reaching for that goal.

Think of a goal as a guideline or road map to get us where we want to go. Many of us have heard the story about the airplane leaving Los Angeles on the way to Hawaii. They have a map; they set the instruments and head off. And yet, they are constantly making course corrections along the way. They don't say, "Oh well, we are one mile off track" and go back. They have a goal to get to Hawaii, they course correct as needed, and they land in Hawaii.

We may have to course correct on our goals. We sometimes need to modify a bit, and that's okay. And having someone we can share this with and hold us accountable can make all the difference. So many times, I get on a coaching call with someone and they say, "I got this done because I knew I was going to be talking to you." Letting ourselves down is easy; it must be, since we have done it so much. However, most of us hold ourselves to a higher standard when we are being accountable to someone else. Call it pride, self-respect, wanting to look good—whatever, it works.

I had no idea at the time how much these changes would impact my life and my health in the next twenty-five years. I fell in love with coaching—both being coached and coaching and supporting others. And these ideas from so many years ago impact what I do every single day now, and I love it.

Bite-Sized Nugget

Not all coaches are created equal. You need one who understands your problem and your needs; it's worth it to shop for the best coach for you!

IN A NUTSHELL

1. Accountability is often the difference between a dream and attaining a goal. Whether it's being held accountable to yourself or a coach, you must make a 100 percent commitment.

2. Baby steps are the essential first steps. Set small goals which you know you can achieve. As the old saying goes: How do you eat an elephant? One bite at a time.

CHAPTER 6

The Optifast Adventure

Why Feast or Famine Doesn't Work

"And the day came when the risk to remain tight in a bud was more painful than the risk it took to blossom."
—Anais Nin

Opting for Optifast like Oprah

With excitement and nervousness, I began my first year of one-on-one coaching to build my real estate business. It's interesting to me when I look back and realize this was also the beginning of my next big diet adventure—Optifast.

Another agent in my office was on the Optifast program. I watched her lose weight, and the change was pretty dramatic. She was consistently losing weight every week. Finally, I decided to ask her about it and see how it worked. All I knew about the program was that Oprah had done it and I had made a point of watching the episode where she did the reveal. She pushed a wheelbarrow onto the stage carrying something that represented the amount of weight she lost, about 65 pounds. Here was a person in real life, who I knew, doing it and having success.

I asked this other agent to tell me about it, how she was liking it and how hard it was. It was very simple, you simply just stopped eating—completely. Instead, you had five shakes a day and two optional faux chicken bouillon soups daily. I said I could not imagine not eating at all and asked if she didn't get hungry. She explained that once you were a few days into the program, your body got used to the diet and you really weren't hungry.

After speaking with her, I decided to take the next step and get more information. We had the same insurance company, and this program was covered. I was skeptical, but by this time my weight had climbed to what was then my all-time high of 269 pounds.

The Adventure of a Lifetime

That same day I called and found my next step was to attend an informational meeting. There were about forty people in the meeting, and I took my normal front-row spot. They offered three different programs: the full fast, a partial fast (you had five shakes a day and one meal), and some kind of eating plan. Being well established as the all-or-nothing girl, I signed up for the full fast.

The full fast was no food—only liquids until you got within ten pounds of your goal weight. At that point you begin to reintroduce foods back into your daily diet. Each session lasted 20 weeks with required weekly two-hour meetings. If you had not reached your goal weight at the end of 20 weeks, you re-upped for 20 more weeks. I knew I was going to be doing several of these 20-week segments. The meetings were to address the psychological reasons for our weight and work on changing mindsets and behaviors around food; in other words, dealing with our "issues" around food. Before we left the meeting, we also had to sign up for a two-part physical to make sure we were healthy enough to do the fast and an appointment with an Optifast staff member to get us started on the program after the release from the doctor. I left the meeting with appointment slips in hand, ready to get this thing started.

After my physical, I met with the Optifast counselor. The information meeting, the counselor appointment, and the actual Optifast weekly meetings were all held in the same building, so each time you were there you saw people checking in for their classes. In the lobby, where the receptionist area was, there were two huge floor scales. You took a slip of paper and placed it in a slot on the side of the scale. When you were on the scale, you pressed a button and your weight was automatically printed on the slip of paper, which we took with us to our class. Much more civilized than the clipboard lady at the end of the line back in high school! It was more like the individual weigh-ins at Weight Watchers, except here only you saw your weight.

My meeting with the counselor included having measurements taken, my body fat percentage measured, the famous "before" photos taken, and choosing an Optifast class. I left with a notebook of all the lessons for the first 20 weeks, with my photos, measurements, and body fat information inside. We also received a textbook. I was all set: I was eager to get started and nervous to see if I would be able to just stop eating.

My first meeting was the next week, Tuesday at 6:30 p.m. My Optifast leader was Robin. Walking in that room the first time was scary; I felt the same as I had when I walked into my first Weight Watchers meeting, except I was now about 70 to 80 pounds heavier. Once again, I was worried about being the fattest person in the room. The room was packed. This was January, after all (New Year's resolutions and all that), and I was about in the middle, weight-wise.

At this meeting, Robin shared a bit about her personal history, her education, and why she taught these classes. I did not feel a sense of rapport with her, but that was not the reason I was there. After she introduced herself, she asked each of us to introduce ourselves and share something about us that had nothing to do with weight. She started with the far side of the room and went around the circle. Because there is no front row in a circular seating arrangement, my new "spot" was the chair next to the door. This seemed like the closest thing to the front row, or maybe I just wanted to be able to make a quick getaway. I really was not able to pay much attention to the other members' introductions, because I was too busy racking my brain trying to think of something to say when it was my turn. When they got to me, I blurted out something like this:

My Entire Life Revolved Around What I Ate and What I Weighed

"My name is Judi. This is my first time doing the Optifast program, and I cannot think of a single thing to say about me that doesn't have something to do with weight. I have spent most of my adult life from the age of twenty gaining weight, losing weight, wondering what diet I was going to do next, wondering what I was going to eat or not eat next, and being constantly disappointed I could not lose weight and keep it off."

Bite-Sized Nugget
Your worth is not determined by a number on the scale. What you weigh is NOT who you are.

As pitiful as that sounded, most things in my life had to do with my weight. Everything in my somewhat warped perspective on my life revolved around my weight. The first week of the program we had to eat "normally" and record what we ate, when we ate, and then turn that log in at our second meeting. After our second meeting, at which we picked up our shakes and our soups, we were ready to start the program. The five shakes were to be spaced two to three hours apart during the day and the soups could be added whenever we wanted.

That next morning, I had my first shake at home. Mixed with water, it wasn't too bad. I put a couple of boxes of shakes in my car trunk along with water and paper cups, and off to work I went. When I got to work, I put another of the shakes into my desk. On my first day I was showing houses to a couple from Los Angeles moving to our area, and I knew we would be out for several hours.

Having Your Food Your Way

It was time for my shake, I told the couple I was with. I explained I had just started a special diet and had to have a shake every three hours, and I asked if they minded. They did not mind, and at our next stop, I opened the trunk, quickly made and drank a shake, and went on to the next house. This incident was pivotal for me in one of my coaching beliefs. Never be embarrassed about the steps you are taking to get healthy. Never apologize for what you are doing or be afraid to ask for what you need. An example is eating a meal in a restaurant and being very clear with the server what you want and how you want it prepared. You are the customer and deserve to have it "your way!"

Being honest about my food choices was a pivotal step in losing the weight. I decided not to be embarrassed about what I was doing and why. Yes, other people could think I was weird, crazy, rude, or all of the above. To be successful, I had to be committed. Over the months as I followed the program, drinking my shakes and forgoing meals became normal and automatic. No one ever ridiculed me, said anything negative, or fired me as their realtor. The clients I worked with became my cheerleaders.

Bite-Sized Nugget

Eat for you! Stop being embarrassed about your special requests, need for healthy food in your car, or any other protocol which helps keeps you on track.

Often, I took clients out to lunch while looking at houses and to dinner to celebrate their new homes. And I learned socializing did not mean I had to eat what they were eating, or at this time in my life, to even eat at all. I would ask for water without ice, add my shake, and drink my shake while they were eating. When my clients ordered coffee, I would ask for hot water and make one of my soups.

As a coach, I hear too often that people are afraid to ask for what they want. They go out with friends and family and are worried about what others think of their food choices. They may worry about feeling different when asking for special food items or preparations. They may also feel pressured to not eat differently and so order food they do not really want to be consuming. My answer is always the same: It doesn't matter what others think of what you are eating—why would they even care? My theory is that your healthy choices make them feel guilty about what they are eating, and they don't want to look bad in comparison to you.

Picture a big bucket of crabs. There are always one or two crabs who seem intent on climbing out of the bucket. They scramble around, trying to inch their way up the side of the bucket, reaching for the top to pull themselves out. While they are working hard to escape the bucket, the rest of the crabs are trying to pull them back in. In the end, no crabs get out.

Some people are like the crabs pulling others back into the bucket. Some people want to keep everyone else in the unhealthy bucket with them. They don't want to get out, so they don't want you to get out either, which makes them feel bad about themselves. When someone says to you, "Why are you ordering that?" or "Why can't you have some of this with us?" picture the bucket of crabs. Don't let others keep you in the bucket. (You could turn the question around and ask them why they are ordering what they did.)

When you decide to get healthy and start making changes in your life, others may feel threatened and may believe your choices are shining a light on their unhealthy choices. They may think you expect them to do the same, and they become very defensive of their choices.

One of my clients has had great success with her weight loss and has created amazing healthy habits for her kids. However, her husband, who has over 100 pounds to lose, doesn't want to change. He tries to sabotage her by bringing unhealthy foods home, refusing to eat the healthy meals she makes, and inviting their kids to join him in eating the unhealthy food. He is the crab trying to keep others (in this case, his family) in the bucket.

IN A NUTSHELL

1. Make the choices that keep you committed to your goal; stop worrying about what others think and how they might perceive you.
2. Climb out of the bucket and don't let other crabs bring you down to their level. Not everyone will celebrate your successful change in habits, as it often highlights their own unhealthy ones.

CHAPTER 7

One Bad Apple Doesn't Spoil the Barrel

How to Stop Feeling Like a Failure

"Even the biggest failure beats the hell out of never trying."
—Anonymous

Becoming a Weight-Loss Rock Star

I nailed it: I was an Optifast rock star, a poster child for the brand. Similar to every diet I had tried before, I was *perfect*.

There's a term for a fear of being imperfect: atelophobia. I share this word with you because perfectionism and the B+

Diet are at odds with each other. You cannot be perfect on this program, nor am I asking you to. Instead, I'm recognizing that every day is life; there are celebrations and sadness, unexpected issues and planned success. However, when you live by healthy rules 85 percent of the time, it results in weight loss.

You can detect my atelophobia when I share that in ten months, not one single bite of solid food passed my lips ... except once. When I had been on the Optifast program for about three or four months, Kevin and I took a couple out to dinner who had just successfully closed escrow on their dream house. I had my shake and my soup. As we were walking out of the restaurant, I picked up a mint from the front desk and automatically popped it into my mouth without even thinking. If I hadn't taken that one mint, I would have been perfect. (See? I hate the fact that I wasn't perfect.) When I realized I had it in my mouth, I actually spat it out and didn't eat it.

Believe it or not, I was never really hungry after the first week. When you stop eating, your body goes into ketosis. Ketosis occurs when you're fasting or on a low carbohydrate diet which causes the body to burn ketones instead of glucose and is the basis of the Keto diet, which I do not recommend. I don't believe it is healthy or sustainable long-term. Don't forget: I was on a medically supervised program with required doctor appointments, tests, and screenings every single week.

The wild part of my fasting was that I started having dreams I was eating. The sensation of eating felt wonderful, and yet I woke up feeling guilty. I didn't want to believe I had goofed and gone off my no-eating plan. I later discovered dreaming about food and eating was a common side effect of fasting.

I started Optifast in January at the very same time I began paying Tim of the Mike Ferry Organization $1,000 per month to build my business. The requirements for each goal (weight loss and revenue) made me commit to a rigorous schedule of when I would drink my shakes and what I would do daily to grow my real estate business.

My real estate business was growing, and in my coaching program, I earned the award for "Most Improved Rookie of the Year." This award meant more to me than any award I had ever received. Adding to the excitement was that I also was invited to be a panelist at the Superstar Retreat in August in Palm Desert. Approximately 2,000 real estate agents would be attending. The interest for the conference was so great that a second retreat was added in October in Naples, Florida. I was invited to speak at that event as well.

So here I was being recognized in August at the real estate conference not only for my business success, but for my weight loss as well. I lost over 100 pounds by the time I hit that stage. It seemed as if more people wanted to talk to me about the weight loss than the real estate!

By October at the next real estate conference, I was almost to my goal of losing 150 pounds. I went shopping for a new outfit to wear on stage for the panel. I bought this amazing three-piece suit, skirt, vest, and long jacket in a platinum color with shimmery silver threads running throughout. It was fabulous.

I had silver shiny nylons and silver pumps. I dubbed that suit my "panelist suit," and every time I wore it, I remembered how proud I was of being chosen to be a panelist. One of my favorite memories is sitting in a director's style chair in that suit and crossing my legs and being able to tuck one behind the other when I did it. (When you are a fat person, crossing your legs, sitting "Indian style," or tucking your legs up under you is difficult, if not impossible.)

Come November, my husband and I were off on a month-long trip to Maui. I had finally reached my goal weight with Optifast in November and started the reintroduction of food the following week. By the time we were ready to leave for our trip, I was finished with shakes and back completely on food. In ten months, I had lost 151.5 pounds, and at the same time I had quadrupled my income from my real estate business.

Amazing coincidence? I don't think so. In both cases, I followed *a very clearly defined plan* and *committed 100 percent*. The weight goal I had chosen and achieved was pretty low—about 12 pounds less than when I got married. Kevin thought I was too thin, but I loved it. No one had ever told me that I was too thin. Thin!

Bite-Sized Nugget

When you are all in with a commitment and a mindset, you will succeed.

Upon my return to San Diego, I remember eating lunch by myself one day at the counter at Mimi's, a chain of cafés. The lady sitting next to me asked how my lunch was (bruschetta), and I said great. She then remarked, "You are so tiny, it probably doesn't matter what you eat." Shocked, I realized how odd that sounded to me. My immediate thought was, "You should have seen me 150 pounds ago." Thank goodness I didn't say it aloud.

From Rock Star to Falling Star

By the following August, I had gained back about 30 to 40 pounds and was terrified of attending the real estate retreat. I was embarrassed about my weight gain. Because Mike Ferry and others had made such a big deal over my weight loss the previous year, I felt I would look like a failure. The year before, I had had so much fun choosing outfits to bring, and this year, not so much. I bought several new suits the month before we went to the retreat. Imagine my horror when we got the hotel and I discovered none of those new suits fit; they were all too small.

I had to face the reality of my weight gain. I had to admit to my friend and roommate that I had to go shopping again. I bought what fit and had to deal with it.

It wasn't just the weight gain but the psychological pain that hurt tremendously. I spent much of the time at the retreat ducking people I did not want to see. I felt sorry for myself, I felt guilty, and I felt like a failure again. These are the deadly thoughts that contributed to my pattern of losing and gaining weight.

Weight Gain Eating at My Confidence

Just as I did with Weight Watchers (WW), I rejoined the Optifast program. Doing it for the second time was harder, just as it was harder to lose the weight the second, third, fourth, and fifth times on WW. Going back to something where I'd been a success felt like a failure. The failure ate away my confidence.

At the beginning of each new group I was in, I did not get to say I was there for the first time. Instead, I had to admit I had been a member before, lost weight, gained some back, and here I was. In my mind, I was telling the group I was a loser.

In my negative perfectionism, each time I rejoined, I wanted to weigh more than the last time I rejoined; this way I could have more to lose, and that would make me more of a success. How convoluted and crazy is that kind of thinking? Remember those big scales I mentioned? One time when rejoining for what felt like the millionth time, I weighed in on the scale holding a full double Big Gulp stealthily by my side. I had weighed it at home and knew it weighed at least 3 pounds. Pretty sad, right?

This pattern of losing/gaining and success/failure has been so destructive in both my weight and my self-image. I judged my self-worth by how I looked in the mirror.

IN A NUTSHELL

1. Make the choices which keep you committed to your goal; stop worrying about others and how they might perceive you.
2. Your worth is not measured by pounds or the mirror; it's measured by how you appreciate and celebrate you!

CHAPTER 8

A Taste of Coaching
The Differentiator Between Dreams and Goals

"Life does not get better by chance, it gets better by change."
—Jim Rohn

For the next several years, my real estate business continued to do well, while my weight went up and down. After Optifast, I did the Lindora program. My best friend had done it, and she was the lightest I had ever seen her. Once again, the diet worked, and I was at my healthy weight, reinforcing my assertion that all diets work. The key question is can you stay with the program for life? As I would learn again and again, the answer was no.

The Joy of Coaching

I had been asked to become a coach for the Mike Ferry Organization, teaching other realtors how to build their businesses. I was really excited about the opportunity. I loved having a coach and thought it would be amazing to *be* a coach, so I said yes. I also signed a noncompete clause preventing me from coaching real estate agents for six months if I stopped working for the Ferry Organization. The coaching took some time away from my own real estate business, but it cemented my belief in the process of coaching, the power of coaching, and the results of coaching.

I had only my own personal experience of being coached as a model to follow. A surprising "aha moment" occurred when I discovered that some of my clients weren't invested in their own results. It was as if my clients wanted me to "will" them across the finish line. Let's be clear: your coach can't want your success more than you do!

Further, the clients who were awarded coaching versus paying out of their pocket had vastly different results. It's similar to hosting an event for free and then finding that over 50 percent didn't show up. Why? Because there was no penalty for not showing up. Good coaching requires accountability and commitment. You must pay to stay.

Bite-Sized Nugget

If you pay for coaching, you stay for coaching. If you pay nothing, the perception is that the value is nothing.

At one point as a real estate coach, I thought I should branch out and become a weight-loss coach. Heck! I had lost and found over 1,500 pounds by that time. I also thought, erroneously, that coaching others would spur my own weight loss—wrong! The mindset is the magic. I couldn't coach others if I didn't believe in myself. I didn't take my own advice when it came to weight loss. As a result, I got heavier, my confidence plummeted, and I quit coaching about weight loss.

Bite-Sized Nugget

Coaching is the difference between dreaming and achieving.

I decided instead of just weight-loss coaching, I would venture into life coaching. I stopped working with Mike Ferry and waited out my noncompete clause. Of course, my first clients were real estate agents because they already knew and loved me.

Not only did I coach my clients to success, but I celebrated with them. Their drive helped me understand the true human potential; if we let go of our fears and decide to do whatever it takes to succeed, we can achieve anything. One unexpected benefit of my coaching was uncovering my love of speaking. A client asked me to speak, and I felt the energy of the room.

At this same time, I felt the first stirrings of wanting to write a book. One of my clients had set a goal to write a book. I coached her, supported her, and was her cheerleader. When that book was published, I'm not sure who was more excited, her or me!

Another one of my clients lived in an oceanfront condo right on the beach. I rented a portion of a room from her and decided this space would be my writing place. I made all of the arrangements; I set up the room with a perfect view, I moved in all of the tools, notebooks, pens, and books. And then, nothing. I couldn't seem to transfer my thoughts onto paper. Oh, I would write a few pages and then I'd lose the drive. Eventually, I found myself in my little rented waterfront space paying money to read about writing and not writing anything. Clearly, this rental wasn't a good investment. For a time, I gave up on my dream of writing a book.

The entire time I was conducting life coaching, I was still working as a real estate agent. Finally, as my coaching business grew, I knew this profession was my passion and I left the real estate business (at the height of the market, which no one does). It was time to do what I loved, not what made the most money. I also discovered the coach's dilemma—if you charge by the hour, you limit your income because there are only so many hours in the day. Although I was fully booked with coaching calls, my current model didn't allow me to boost my income.

I attended an event in Berkeley with Marcia Wieder, America's Dream Coach, who was offering Dream Coach University. We would be spending six days being taught by Marcia and becoming Certified Dream Coaches. I was so excited to go. Little did I realize that two people who I met at this event would play a big role in shaping the direction of my life.

One of these people was Joan, who was a coach like me. She understood the limited income dilemma if your only revenue source is charging by the hour. As a result, we created products which could earn residual income—sell the same product over and over again.

Bite-Sized Nugget
Trading hours for dollars is a losing and limiting proposition. Look at selling products or services to a group to boost your reputation and income.

Networking Was Working to Grow My Reach and Reputation

Joan also introduced me to the DSWA (Direct Selling Women's Alliance). Founded in 2001, it's an association devoted to getting women in direct selling to succeed. It provides resources, trainings, and tools to its members. Although I hadn't heard of it nor had I joined, Joan suggested we join as a Corporate Member. Her initial thought was that we would be able to place our coaching program in their online store. It would be a great way to boost our visibility and sales.

However, it didn't turn out like that. Our success with DSWA was better than we could have imagined. Almost instantaneously, we were invited to lead teleclasses. I was loving it because I was utilizing both my coaching and speaking gifts.

Three days after joining, I received a phone call from Grace, one of the three founding members of the organization. She invited me to meet Nikki, the president, for dinner when she came to San Diego the next week. I said yes, of course!

My conversation with Nikki that night was life-changing for me. Nikki helped me understand the power of direct selling: how to create residual income and support others doing the same. I left that dinner knowing I had to join a direct selling organization.

Similar to you, I was familiar with Amway (negative perception), Tupperware, Mary Kay, and even Avon. However, I didn't really understand the magnitude of the industry and its impact on the economy. The women Nikki told me about pursued their careers with a vengeance. They treated it like the business that it was, not a mere hobby.

Within a few days after the monumental dinner with Nikki, one of the founders offered me a role in the organization. My first project was to work on the sequel to the book *Build It Big*. This book became a textbook of the industry, sharing insights from successful sales leaders. It was so successful that my job was to interview the stars of the industry for *More Build It Big*.

Since all of the featured sales representatives had achieved either the first or second spots in sales for their companies, I earned an unofficial PhD in direct selling. I soaked up their wisdom like a baby sponge.

I also started exploring direct selling opportunities, determined to find the right fit. I began exploring direct selling companies, and my number-one criterion was they had to provide a product I loved and believed in completely.

I found a new company offering weight-loss solutions which were good and not "magic answers" and decided to join. Next step was to find the right sponsor. When I was doing the interviews for *More Build It Big*, the people I talked to shared what a key tool for success the right sponsor could be.

I searched and found several current reps and set up interviews with them. I met Cori and liked her right away, and I trusted her and her commitment to helping me succeed in the business.

Cori was a great teacher, and we had rapport right off the bat. I explained my weight-loss history and shared that I wanted to embrace the program and products and demonstrate to myself and my future customers it could be done. I started the program, the company, and again another program to lose weight. Without really knowing what I was doing, I was slowly growing my business, signing up customers and distributors, and had no idea what to do with them next. Once again, I was not doing very well with my weight loss. In essence, I liked the business model of network marketing, but didn't make the full commitment to the program. I was selling a program in which I wasn't fully invested. Similar to other efforts, I started an adventure, but quit too early. As you'll see later, I only enjoyed financial and wellness success with Beachbody when I was "all in."

Buying Team Women

When I first met Milan, I was still working in real estate. She was a star in the direct selling industry, and I later learned that she never asked me to join her because she assumed I wasn't interested. In other words, because I was successful in real estate, she assumed other opportunities were closed. Ironically, what I've learned from direct selling is that if you're successful in one area, you'll also be successful in another area.

Her latest venture was turning a wine club company into a direct sales company hosting in-home wine-tasting parties, appropriately named Got Great Wine. This time when she asked, I answered with a resounding "yes!" I also thought it was a good fit, because I enjoyed wine and here was an opportunity not tied to weight loss. My success would not depend on whether or not I was losing weight. While I loved this business, the wine took its toll, leading me to an all-time highest weight of 350+ pounds.

Bite-Sized Nugget

Stop making assumptions. Think of asking someone to join you on a journey as an exclusive invitation.

Again, because of my enthusiasm, I was able to start growing this business. Seriously, it was wine, how hard could it be?
When I was interviewing all of those top income earners for
the book *More Build It Big,* they all shared that one of the best
ways to grow your business was to network. And being clueless,
I thought that meant hooking two computers together! They
explained it was going out and meeting other business owners,
making a connection, and building a relationship.

Needless to say, I therefore started attending local networking meetings. There were many in my area, such as BNI, LeTip,
Ali Lassen Leads, and even chamber of commerce meetings.
While I was in a great business and most people were interested
in wine, none of them seemed exactly the right fit for me. Then
I found a group called Team Women, which had a few chapters, but none in my area. I talked to the owner and asked if I
could open a chapter in Carlsbad, and I did. At my first meeting, there were two of us there. I did wine tastings, and she sold
jewelry. I bought a pair of earrings, and she booked my very first
wine-tasting party.

We each committed to bring a guest to the following meeting. There were four of us at the next meeting, eight at the meeting after that, and soon we had over 25 members. I was having
so much fun with this business that I was spending about half
of my time working my wine business and the other half looking for Team Women members. I had requests from people in
other areas for chapters, and within six weeks I had opened an
astounding eight chapters in San Diego! I was also the acting
president in each new chapter until someone else could step into

that role. Team Women continued to grow, and three months later I bought the company. I really dove in then, and within three years, we had 150 chapters across the US and Canada.

Now I had two full-time businesses: Team Women and the wine business. I spent three out of four weeks traveling to open new chapters, and every time I had a new wine consultant somewhere, we opened a new chapter for them. Both businesses were doing great. I was hosting wine tastings, drinking a lot of wine, eating in hotels, and my weight continued to rise.

Business Goals at the Expense of Weight-Loss Goals

With all of the travel, I experienced for the first time the embarrassment of having to ask for a seat belt extender. Mortifying! Although the flight attendants acted as if it was no big deal, my fellow passengers looked at me with pity. Or so I thought. I so dreaded the exchange about requesting an extender, I began taking an extender with me in my purse. It was a low point for me. I was blocking my feelings. I had no commitment to lose the weight.

IN A NUTSHELL

1. Get a coach—now! It truly determines whether or not you reach your goals. I would be honored to coach you. Please reach out to me for how to work together.
2. Weight loss is a way of life. Never derail your personal goals (weight loss) for professional goals. A healthy life is one that embraces all of you.
3. When it comes to networking, find your tribe. Not all organizations are a good fit for you. Try many before settling on a group.

CHAPTER 9

Fed Up

Taking the First Step
with Beachbody

"Don't just talk about what you want to accomplish. Make it happen." —Unknown

Everything was going along fine in my life. I was opening new chapters for Team Women and I was selling wine. In short, life was great as long as I overlooked the fact that I was more than 175 pounds overweight! I had given up on ever reaching and maintaining a healthy weight. Too many successes followed by failures had eroded any confidence I once had. I didn't believe I could lose the weight. I decided it was easier to give up and stop trying than to disappoint myself over and over again.

Giving Up Isn't an Option

I accepted that my way of life and weight were going to stay the way they were ... until my friend Milan called me. She had left the wine business, remarried, and was enjoying a semi-retirement with her new husband (also a Kevin). She told me that she and Kevin were thinking of joining a company that had piqued their interest. They had met with one of the founders, learned about his vision for the company with them, and had become excited about the possibilities. She told me a bit about the company and asked me to check it out. I wished her well and promptly forgot about it.

A few weeks later, she called me back and asked if I'd had a chance to check out the company. I confessed that I had not made the time. Her Kevin had joined the corporate side of the company, and she was going to join the selling side of the business. All of her years of experience had been on the corporate side, so she was excited to see how the "other side" lived. She asked me again to check out the company website. I was happy for her and wished her well again; then I went on with what I was doing.

When she called again, this time the light went on. I pointedly asked her, "Are you trying to recruit me for this company?" She admitted she was. When I asked her why she had not just said that to begin with, she explained she was concerned because she knew how well I was doing with the wine business she had gotten me into, and I was also busy with Team Women. However, she remembered when she had assumed I was too successful to be interested in an opportunity; she had committed to not make that mistake again, and that was why she was calling.

I asked her to tell me more about the company with the prospect of me joining her. The company, Beachbody, had been selling in-home workout programs very successfully for years. A community of loyal customers had grown organically. Within this community, customers were supporting other customers, encouraging them to work out, and eat right. Customers were consistently experiencing solid weight loss and health successes. People started mailing in their before-and-after photos to the company, sharing their stories and expressing their gratitude for how their lives had changed.

Milan asked me to attend the "Founders Meeting" of Beachbody, which was coming up quickly. This meeting was the kickoff for their coaching program. They were formalizing this organic community and creating a team of coaches to support customers who purchased their programs.

Milan explained to me that approximately forty people would be attending the meeting. Most of these people were active participants of the program and had experienced transformations. They were living, breathing examples of how the products worked. Those of us who were not experienced with the program were invited to join because we understood the business model and believed in it. Those who invited us thought our business perspectives would make us great coaches. I asked Milan very directly if I would be the fattest person there. She answered honestly, probably yes.

Hearing that, I made up my mind that there was no way I wanted to attend. It was already hurtful being the fattest person in the room in day-to-day life. The last thing I wanted was to be that person in a room full of fitness fanatics, so I said no.

Becoming One of the First Forty Beachbody Coaches

Thank goodness Milan did not give up on me. She gave me all the details. The meeting was going to be held over a weekend, and Beachbody was picking up the tab for three nights at the Beverly Wilshire Hotel, just off Rodeo Drive. This hotel is where most of my all-time favorite movie *Pretty Woman* with Richard Gere and Julia Roberts was filmed. I can't tell you how many times I have watched it. The chance to spend three nights free at this hotel on my birthday weekend was a tantalizing draw.

Just as I had when mulling over whether to move to Hawaii, I thought through what was the worst thing that could happen if I went to the Founders Meeting weekend. I decided the worst thing that could happen was that I would hate the event, experience some embarrassment, and then never have to think about it again.

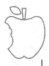

Bite-Sized Nugget

Remember the 1971 Alka-Seltzer slogan "Try it, you'll like it"? Think of this catchphrase as you try new foods and new ways of thinking.

A reception was scheduled for Thursday evening. On Friday evening, Beachbody was taking us all out to dinner. Milan and Kevin had set up a dinner with the president of the coaching side of the business for eight of us at CUT, the fancy new restaurant owned by Wolfgang Puck. Okay, what the heck, I thought—and decided to go.

On the night of the dinner, I met my husband at the bar—the one made famous in *Pretty Woman*, where Richard Gere met Julia Roberts to take her to the opera and she was wearing that perfect red dress. Kevin walked in carrying a bouquet of red roses for my birthday.

When we meandered off to the Founder's reception, I met corporate employees and participants. No one shunned me or made me feel bad for being there; several attendees took time to share their amazing stories with me. One man had lost over 100 pounds; another woman had lost 85 pounds. Stories like these sparked a desire to join this amazing team. Please understand that at the time, the coaching side of the business was called Million Dollar Body. The name was intimidating for someone like me with so much weight to lose.

The first real friend I made at Beachbody was Michael Neimand, who was a vice president. He was excited about the launch. I asked him why the coaching business was called Million Dollar Body. He explained it was because in the first year of operation for the coaching business, Beachbody would be awarding $1,000,000.00 in prize money to people for their weight loss and fitness successes. Michael spent over an hour chatting with me that evening, and I am sure he has no idea how much that meant to me when I felt like a fraud for even being there.

On the morning of my birthday, the official meeting was launched. I took my normal front-row aisle seat and sat there nervous and not sure what to expect. Kevin and Milan were there with another couple they had invited from the wine business. When the president opened the meeting, he said there was something they had to do before the meeting started. Imagine my shock when they sang "Happy Birthday" to me! I found myself really warming up to this company and getting good vibes.

During the day, many of the executives spoke. When Carl Daikeler, President of Beachbody, shared his vision and passion, I was hooked. Here was a man who believed in his company's ability to help solve the obesity problem in America. He was on a mission to do everything he could to make it happen.

Several of the celebrity trainers also spoke to us that day, including Tony Horton, the creator of Power 90 and P90X, and Kathy Smith, who had been in the fitness industry for years. When Kathy took the stage, she said she wanted someone to come up on stage with her and pointed to me. I was panicked. Here I was weighing over 300 pounds standing next to a beautiful, thin, fit role model. In truth, I don't remember what she said, but I remember that she held my hand the whole time she spoke. As she held my hand, I felt a stirring of hope. I thought, "Maybe I really can do this."

I calculated how much weight I would need to lose to reach a normal weight, not even my dream weight. It came to 200 pounds. I wondered if I were setting myself up to be disappointed again.

As Carl talked about how the coaching would work, I was impressed by his commitment and fearful of my own ability to do something I had failed at over and over. The day ended and we all went to dinner, where we had a chance to get to know each other better.

Saturday morning, day two, was to be the day we decided if we were going to join Beachbody and be part of the launch scheduled for December 29, just two weeks away. I knew I loved coaching, but also had little faith in myself; however, I believed the opportunity to share my struggles and challenges might be useful to those I would be coaching.

I thought about my other direct selling experiences, from the DSA to the wine business to Team Women. In hindsight, of course, I wish I had chosen opportunities more in alignment with my goals. As I mentioned, the wine business was at odds with my weight-loss vision, and Team Women kept me on the road, making it more difficult to make good decisions.

However, here was an opportunity to not only get in on the ground floor of a new business, but to share with others my journey with others and support them. I said yes!

The Beginning of Believing

My reasons for saying yes and becoming a coach are the same today as they were that day many years ago. As a coach, when I encouraged others to work out, eat better, and make healthier choices, I had to do the same. Doing anything else would not be acting with integrity or authenticity.

I knew supporting and coaching others had become my passion. I wanted to motivate and encourage my clients to achieve accomplishments they didn't realize they were capable of. I liked holding the "faith" for them. I understood their lack of confidence, and I remembered one of the most important things, Tim, my real estate coach said to me: "If you had half the faith in you that I have in you, you would be unstoppable." That was the message I wanted to share with others.

The opportunity to get paid to do what I loved and would do for free was simply amazing. I signed on the dotted line, and off we went for a tour of the Beachbody offices. Before leaving, I committed to Carl that I was going to do this program and that I planned to lose 200 pounds.

We piled into a bus, so excited about the journey we were going to be undertaking. It is amazing looking back to realize how small the Million Dollar Body business was then. The company had about forty employees and there we were, the first forty coaches. Only one person didn't commit to Beachbody that day.

On the tour, the mission came alive. The walls were covered with before-and-after photos of customers with their stories. They were real. It was apparent these were not studio shots; they were photos customers had taken and wanted to share. The photos evoked a sense of possibility and excitement in every-one. At the end of the tour, the formal meetings were over; we were coaches and wondered what was next.

Bite-Sized Nugget

Find a coach who embraces this philosophy about you: If you had half the faith in you that I have in you, you would be unstoppable.

My stretch goal was to lose enough weight to fit into the wedding dress I wore when Kevin and I got married. I liked having a goal that was not based on a number on a scale. I chose December 29 as the day I was going to start my workout program and had chosen Power 90. I had been told it was a great entry-level program that I could modify as needed.

To be clear, I had never done any kind of official workout program. I had run in the past, played racquetball, had tried a few 30-minute circuit training programs, and that was about it. I had bought treadmills, an elliptical machine, and an exercise bike. I had probably used each of these machines no more than three times. My treadmill had become the laughable place to hang clothes. Working out was all new to me. I had loved running when I did it, had fun with racquetball when we played, and once, Kevin and I had walked eight miles for the March of Dimes, and couldn't move for a week.

So, on December 29, I put the video in and attempted the workout. I had never really been a fan of exercise for the purpose of just working out. Part of it could be due to how totally uncoordinated I am; well, "klutz" is a better way to describe it. For example, once I stood on a curb, wearing a pair of wedge sandals, talking to Kevin who was getting things out of the car. I was just standing there, lost my balance, fell into the gutter, and broke not one but *both* ankles. So, you can see why I wasn't totally into exercise.

The video was about 28 minutes long, and I did the best I could. I thought I was literally going to die. I weighed in at 319.75 pounds at 5 feet 4 inches. I did not know about warming up or how to prepare for a workout. The next day, I did the next workout, injured my back, and had a hard time getting up off the floor. Two days into working out and I was already out with an injury. I could barely walk and ended up having to visit the chiropractor three times. This was not an auspicious start to my new fitness business.

Meanwhile, the launch of the Million Dollar Body was delayed a few times while they worked on computer issues. Over the next few months, there were several false starts, and the new site did not officially launch until April 2007. And then we were open!

During the first year, I won one of the monthly contests for my approximately 50-pound weight loss and also achieved one of the Top Coach slots for 2007. My weight loss and sales also earned me a spot on the Top Coach Trip to Maui.

Here I was celebrating my role as a great coach, yet my weight was still out of control. Yes, I was down 50 pounds, but I was still the only overweight team member going. My mindset was that I was going to enjoy my trip anyway. When we got to the airport, they were having a "sale" on first-class upgrades, and Kevin and I upgraded in a heartbeat. Sheer bliss!

We stayed at the Hyatt Regency in Wailea and had a spectacular oceanfront room. The first night, Beachbody hosted a reception. Carl handed out envelopes with $100 of spending money. We also got to choose an activity. Kevin golfed and I opted for a foot massage and pedicure.

There were daily workouts on the beach with Tony Horton. One day in the elevator on our way to the workout, the elevator was filled with coaches and other hotel guests. A little boy, around 8 or 9 years old, looked at me, turned to his mom and asked, "Why is that lady so fat?" You could have heard a pin drop in the embarrassed silence of that elevator. The mom quickly apologized, and I am sure I must have told her it was all right. But inside I was not all right because I felt I had no one but myself to blame.

As would become clear to me throughout my years of weight-loss struggle, I had to own my weight. I didn't weigh over 300 pounds because I ate too many bananas or too much broccoli. I overindulged often, and the results were clearly visible to me and everyone else.

IN A NUTSHELL

1. Any day is a good day to start your new journey. It doesn't matter if you're the heaviest person in the room or on a trip. Welcome a new way of thinking.
2. Yes, you can! You are never too old or too fat to start. Believe.

CHAPTER 10

I Can't Believe I Ate the Whole Thing

Giving Up on the All-or-Nothing Mindset

"You may be disappointed if you fail, but you are doomed if you don't try." —Beverly Sills

For the next several years, I divided my time and mindset between three businesses: wine, Team Women, and Beachbody. I fooled myself into thinking I was great at running all of them. What I learned is that when you are not 100 percent committed to something, you are robbing yourself of doing the best job you can.

Bite-Sized Nugget

100 percent commitment is the secret ingredient for success.

Multitasking Means Doing Everything Poorly!

I told myself I could do all three jobs, and it was simply not true. In short, I had again embraced my typical overachiever mindset and perfectionist thinking.

I was traveling so much with Team Women that its success was coming at the expense of the wine business. The wine business required conducting tastings to sign up new members. Plus, it required training of new team members. I wasn't spending the time necessary to truly grow the wine business.

Team Women was growing and adding new chapters all the time. The membership fees charged were just enough to cover the costs of maintaining the business expenses. As our membership and income grew, so did the need for support and the costs associated with that growth. So basically, the business sustained itself, but there were no profits. Kevin was always asking me to do a profit-and-loss statement. I resisted because I loved the idea of helping women grow their businesses and did not want to face the fact that it might not be a sustainable business model, nor would it create the freedom I wanted in my life.

Shall we talk about my third business, Beachbody? I poured myself into Team Women and wine so that I could avoid

Beachbody. I wasn't exercising, so my personal goals and business goals weren't in alignment.

As the second annual summit rolled around, I bought a ticket. And then I canceled. I chickened out. As you'll recall, I committed to Carl that I would lose 200 pounds and fit into my wedding dress. I had lost about 20–25 pounds. I didn't want to show up as the Beachbody coach who had so much weight to lose and looked exactly the same as the year before.

Let me tell you that not attending that Beachbody summit is something that I still regret today. Coaching = accountability. Perhaps if I had attended, I would have shifted my mindset sooner. Perhaps I would have had a life-changing moment. Perhaps I would have met the perfect friend. I missed out on all those possibilities because I couldn't face the truth of my situation.

Bite-Sized Nugget
You have to face your problem in order to solve it.

Finally, I Stuck to It!

I was starting to develop a business multiple personality disorder. When someone asked what I did, I had to decide which business I was going to mention and then think about what I was going to say. I was really torn between the three businesses; it showed in my inability to be completely committed to any of them.

The saving grace is that I had not given up on myself. The number-one reason I became a coach was for personal accountability. I had tried workouts from most of the Beachbody programs, but had never completed any program.

I combined my businesses somewhat when I rented office space for Team Women and also used the office for Weekly Fit Clubs. Every week, I gave a short presentation on Beachbody, and then all attendees were invited to stay and join me for the specific workout we were doing for that week. After the workout, participants were offered a protein shake. Weighing in was optional.

At the same time, I decided I was going to finally start and finish an exercise program, no matter what. I choose Kathy Smith, Project You, Type 2. (Don't forget that this was the same exercise guru who had called me up on stage during the inaugural Beachbody meeting.) This was a Beachbody program recommended for beginners, and it was 90 days long. Kevin agreed to do it with me, and we began. The workouts were six days a week and increased in difficulty and duration.

It was tough, but we kept going anyway. Surprisingly, I began losing weight every week. And while I would never become coordinated, some of the moves became easier. I remember the day the workout ended and I said, "Already?" I shocked myself. I was learning that if you just keep doing something, it doesn't get easier—you get better. I was amazed at myself. During the 90-day program I had a problem with one of my knees for a few weeks. In the past, this minor injury would have been the perfect excuse to quit. This time, instead of quitting, I modified the routine and just kept going. We finished the program. I was so proud of us. I had stuck to a program for 90 days, lost weight, and improved my ability to work out.

Completing that program was a milestone for me.

Another shift came when we earned a trip to Costa Rica through the wine business. We were going to be staying in a luxury resort on the ocean in an all-inclusive resort, all expenses paid. This would be our first time in Central America. Exciting!

As more details of the trip were shared, I learned one of our excursions involved zip-lining in the mountain rain forest. I experienced a one-two punch: elated at the possibility and disappointed that I might be too heavy to do it. I called the company in Costa Rica and asked what the weight limit was for zip-lining. For a few seconds I was excited when they said there was no weight limit; but then they mentioned the only restriction was a maximum waist size because of the safety harnesses. Whatever number they uttered, I only remembered that my waist was bigger than that, which meant no zip-lining for me. It was a horrible, depressing feeling to know that I had allowed my weight to be in charge of my life.

Giving Up on the
All-or-Nothing Mindset

After that huge disappointment with the zip line, I signed up for a four-week, one-on-one coaching program with a person who specialized in eating. We specifically talked about my upcoming trip to Costa Rica and a few healthy habits I should pack with me on the trip. She was the person who introduced me to coconut water (which I still love), and I added several boxes in my bags to take with me.

The most important lesson I took away from these sessions had nothing to do with food and more to do with mindset. I believe that my need to be perfect had always been my biggest stumbling block. If I could not be the best, I committed to be the worst. Any misstep or poor choice meant I was a failure and that I had to quit and start over. This lesson was my first step toward dipping my toe into the waters of nonperfection.

My coach suggested that I make informed choices while I was at this all-inclusive resort, not rigid choices. If there was a food I wanted to try, try it. Tasting something did not have to mean I would eat all of it. Really?

It was the beginning of the end of my all-or-nothing approach to food. Food is no longer good or bad food; it's just food! The B+ Diet means that most of the time, approximately 85% (B+), if you choose healthy foods, you will lose weight; you are in control.

Bite-Sized Nugget
There is only food. There are no good foods or bad foods, only choices.

In previous weight-loss programs, I'd been taught that there were foods which were okay to eat and others which were not.

For example, take potato chips—I'd always loved potato chips, and you don't have to be a rocket scientist to know they have no redeeming value as a food. There is nothing healthy about them, and they provide zero nutritional value. In my mind, therefore, they were completely off-limits. It was as if I were an alcoholic: eating just one meant that I had slipped off the program and was a failure. Further, since I believed that I would never "be allowed" to have chips again on a "diet," I must make the most of it and eat the entire bag! This is the mindset that was wrong!

My new coach opened my eyes to the fact that if I really wanted something, I should take *one* bite. If it wasn't great or didn't live up to my expectations, I shouldn't waste any more calories on it. If the food was great, I was to tell myself I could enjoy three bites by eating slowly, savoring each bite. She explained that after three bites, the taste would not get better; it would just be more of the same. So, three and done!

When we went to Costa Rica, I practiced this new philosophy. One of our favorite lunch restaurants there served up a great veggie burger. It came with sweet potato fries. French fries are right up there with chips in my top unhealthy foods. So, when I saw sweet potato fries versus regular fries, I just looked at them and didn't have a bite. On our second visit there, I put my theory to the test. I tried one of the sweet potato fries. It was good, but not as good as regular fries, so I didn't eat more than the one fry. On the third visit, I substituted regular fries. Again, I had one fry. They were certainly better than the sweet potato fries, but not phenomenal. I didn't eat any more. They weren't worthy of more bites and calories to me. Wow! This first step was a monumental one on my road to recovery from perfectionism. One bite doesn't mean that I am a failure or that I "blew my diet." I simply had one fry. And I didn't eat the whole plate. Good for me!

I then applied this theory to dinner. Every night we tried a different restaurant at the resort, giving my husband and me a good taste of variety. At the end of the meal, I'd order one dessert and have one bite. If it was worthy, I would savor three bites. What happened was that I didn't think any of the desserts during the entire week were worthy of three bites. The end result? I came home from Costa Rica 5.5 pounds lighter.

IN A NUTSHELL

1. Today is the perfect day to release the all-or-nothing approach to food. If you have one bite and that's it, you didn't fail; you succeeded! Good for you for not finishing the entire bag, box, or tub.
2. Food is fuel; it is not good or bad, but food. Get released from all of those "old school" thoughts by having one bite of something and then move on.

CHAPTER 11

Half-Baked

How I Learned to Focus

"If you care enough for the result, you will almost always attain it." —William James

I am a big believer in personal development, coaching, and constantly working to learn and improve my skills in business. I had been a longtime follower of Ali Brown, formerly known as the E-zine Queen, and loved watching her success grow. Kevin and I attended a two-day event she hosted where she unveiled the mastermind program she was offering the following year. There were two levels to choose from: $100,000 and $15,000. Since the first ($100k!) was completely out of my price range, I joyfully nabbed the second option.

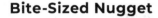

> **Bite-Sized Nugget**
> Great coaches recognize that they too need coaching.

Jack of All Businesses, Master of None

The program included materials, group coaching calls, and several retreats. At the first retreat, I spoke to James, who was co-facilitating with Ali. My question was, "Will this program serve me if I have three businesses and am totally confused about where to focus?" Since James was an employee, he had every vested interest in selling me the idea that the program would benefit me. At the next event, just like other events and trainings I participated in, every time I heard a great idea, I was both excited and confused. I wanted to implement the idea immediately to see how it would work, but I couldn't determine in which business to use it: Team Women, Got Great Wine, or Beachbody.

For the first month of the coaching program, I attended all the calls. Instead of implementing anything, I was frozen. Three months into the program, we had our first three-day retreat, which was filled with amazing women. As I listened to the successes they were having with the program, I realized I was wasting my time, money, and my life by not having a central focus in my business. This lack of focus spilled over into my personal life.

Giving Up the Wine Biz
and Team Women

I looked at my wine business as my "fun" business. Everyone had fun, including me. It was easy to get people interested. I was earning cool trips and had been to New Orleans, Costa Rica, Barcelona, and Paris. Although it was in conflict with my health goals, it was fun to do and fun to talk about; Kevin and I loved it.

Team Women was more about giving back than a profitable business. Perhaps it even was more like a philanthropic enterprise because there was no profit, and all income went right back into the business. The reward to me was being able to provide a way for women to grow their businesses. The coach in me loved being able to provide the means for members to grow and prosper.

Bite-Sized Nugget
There's a huge difference between a business and a hobby. If you enter into business, treat it like one and give it love.

Beachbody, which got the least attention, was what I needed most in my life. I avoided focusing on this business, because if I did, I would have to face the reality of my weight. I mastered avoiding mirrors or only seeing myself from the neck up. In short, I had myopic vision, seeing only what I wanted to see.

Making Tough but Correct Decisions

Thinking back to the retreat, I remember all of the attendees seemed so passionate and focused on what they were doing. I wanted that fire! I just did not know how to get it.

On the second day, Ali went around the room and asked each of us to share what our biggest takeaway from the first day and a half had been. Without even thinking about it, I stood up and said, "What I have realized is without a total focus on one thing, everything is at a level of mediocrity; nothing gets done perfectly. I became a coach because I did not want to give up on myself and my goal to reach and maintain a healthy weight. Without my health, nothing else matters. When I leave this event, I am stepping down from my director position with my wine business, selling Team Women, and focusing 100 percent on Beachbody going forward." Whoa!

Shocked, I sat down and knew the words I had uttered aloud were correct. I had made the right decision—not the easiest decision, but the right one. It felt good and I felt a sense of relief, freedom, and purpose. It wouldn't be easy to let go of my other two businesses, which I loved and had grown and nurtured for years, but it was time to take a stand for me.

There are those times in your life when the universe conspires to show you that you have made the right decision. One of the women sitting at the table with me said she would like to speak with me about buying Team Women. Pretty amazing, right?

The next several months were spent arranging the sale of Team Women. The experience was both gut-wrenching and heartbreaking. Team Women forged friendships across the country; it was inspiring and like my baby that I had nurtured from birth. Yet I knew selling it was the right thing to do.

It was a bit easier to let go of my wine business. I still supported my team when they needed it, but I no longer conducted wine tastings or promoted the business. The friendships I had made were precious. In fact, one of my first wine consultants later joined me at Beachbody. Today, almost fifteen years later, she is the top coach on my team.

IN A NUTSHELL

1. One of the reasons it took me almost my entire adult life to reach my goal of losing the 220+ pounds was my lack of focus. I focused on the easy and fun businesses (wine and women) and avoided the true problem in my life—my weight.

2. I never would have achieved my weight loss, mindset shift, and business success without having paid for coaching with Ali Brown's team. Just because you are a coach doesn't negate the value of having an outsider's perspective as *your* coach.

CHAPTER 12

Eating My Words
Living and Acting Like a Fitness Coach

"Looking after my health today gives me a better hope for tomorrow." —Anne Wilson Schaef

Committed to Beachbody

Since I had sold Team Woman and shed Got Great Wine, it was time for the hard part—focusing on Beachbody and me. In the fairy-tale version of this story, I would tell you I magically achieved every goal, every week the weight fell off my body, and I lived happily ever after. Wrong!

I was still me, the Queen of the Weight Lost-and-Found Department. My weight continued to go up and down, and it was still embarrassing to admit I was a weight-loss and fitness coach when I looked the way I did. I'll never forget how one guy looked me up and down when I told him what business I was in. He asked unbelievingly, "Did you used to be even bigger than you are now?" Hurt, embarrassed, and shocked, I said, "Yes, and I have already lost 30 pounds." What I really wanted to say was, "Yes, and I can always lose more weight, but you will always be rude."

I re-engaged with Beachbody and committed to not giving up, no matter what. I never missed another summit and still regret letting my embarrassment keep me from attending the second one.

In 2009, I had been doing well on my weight loss and had set a goal of being 100 pounds down by the summit. The morning we left, I was down 99.75 pounds. I had missed my goal by 0.25 pound. So instead of celebrating an almost 100-pound weight loss, I focused on the fact that I had missed my goal. I felt like a failure.

If one of my clients had told me they had lost 99.75 pounds with a goal of 100, I would have cheered them on from the rooftops and told them that it was an amazing accomplishment. If I had just kept going, I am sure that 0.25 would have been gone in just a few days.

At the summit, I had been asked to speak on stage and share the strategies which allowed me to achieve Success Club 17 months in a row. I had earned the newly formed title of Success Club All-Star. So here I was being lauded for my accomplishments, and yet all I could do was wallow in my pity of disappointment. As you'll read later, this story is one of the reasons that I became a big fan of celebrating every victory, including non-scale achievements. "Non-scale Victories" (often shortened to NSV) are the benefits of your life choices beyond the scale. It could be going up a flight of steps without huffing and puffing, putting on a pair of jeans that have been too small for years, or easily sitting cross-legged.

Fighting Failure—Again!

After the summit, feeling like a failure, I got off track again. I had lost my confidence, and as a result, I was gaining back the weight. Over the next six to eight months, I allowed myself to regain 50 of those "almost" 100 pounds that I had initially lost.

One of the most embarrassing and mortifying events of my Beachbody business occurred at a leadership event. We were at a hotel in Dana Point, California, and the opening reception was held out on a big lawn. There were round tables with wooden chairs that were sinking a bit into the grass, which made them hard to move. Sitting there, I tried to move my chair to one side so I could get up. Instead of moving, the chair broke and I ended up splayed across the grass with the broken chair in pieces around me. I now knew what it felt like to wish the earth would just swallow me up. Everyone was so nice, almost embarrassingly so, talking about the crummy chairs, etc. Someone took away the broken chair, someone grabbed another chair, and I got up. All I could think of was what everyone must be thinking: here's a fat lady at a health conference and she doesn't even fit into a chair. Writing this now, the pain is just as real. I was horrified that my actions led to me being so heavy. It was a feeling of regret just like when I had consumed eight orders of onion rings and stood in the shower to ignore my neighbor. I didn't want to face the music ... or my neighbor.

Fast-forward a few years to Summit 2015 in Nashville, Tennessee. Again, I really did not want to be there because I was embarrassed to show up as a fitness coach carrying so much weight. Worse, I now weighed 30 pounds more than I had after being celebrated for my almost 100-pound weight loss!

Two things made me attend the summit: one, my regret over missing the second summit and not wanting to make that same mistake twice. The second reason I went was because so many of my great team members were going. I wanted to see and meet them in person and cheer them on.

One of the keynote speakers was Simon Sinek, the author of *Start with Why*. He talked about something called the celery test, and it resonated with me. If, for example, you say you are committed to being healthy, check your shopping cart. Is it filled with celery or cookies? His point being that you must ensure that your actions are congruent with your goals. I got this!

Bite-Sized Nugget
Your actions must be congruent with your goals.

The Ultimate Result—
Starting and Completing a Goal

I told Kevin I was going to do my own celery test. When we got home, I asked him to create a chart where I could track daily if my actions were congruent with my stated goal. In 17 months, it would be my birthday and my ten-year anniversary as a Beachbody coach. I decided to set a goal of reaching my ideal weight by my birthday and my anniversary on December 15, 2016. (As I sit here editing this, it is March 2021.)

Kevin was on board with my goals and lovingly explained that of course I should be at goal weight after being a Beachbody coach for ten years! I committed to a reset program. It is an extremely specific meal program requiring cooking, and best of all to me, no exercising. With a beautiful smile, my husband said he would join me on this reset program.

I was committed to finishing all 21 days of this program. Even though it required cooking, I embraced it. Although my mom was a good cook, her cooking would never be described as healthy. Perhaps I subconsciously become a rebel, turning my nose up at the thought of cooking.

I was nervous about this new program, because with two failures behind me, I did not have any confidence that I could commit and succeed at a goal. Not only did I have Kevin joining me on this journey, but a customer joined me too. At the end of the 21 days, Kevin had lost 14 pounds, I had lost 14.5 pounds, and my customer had also lost 14 pounds. Note here the elements which helped me succeed are a core part of the B+ mindset: goal setting, tracking, and accountability. Was it surprising then that I had finally started a program and finished it?

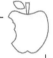

Bite-Sized Nugget
Relish and celebrate every accomplishment—big or small.

Mastering New Food and Life Skills

In addition to being excited about completing the reset, I also began to learn a few new skills:

- Planning meals in advance and making a grocery list from the plan.
- Going grocery shopping and sticking to my list, not what looked good or tempting.
- Figuring out how to make the meal so that all dishes were ready at the same time.
- Prepping ingredients (onions, carrots, celery, etc.) in advance so putting meals together was easy.

I know these new competencies might sound a bit simplistic or elementary to many of you. I was not a big cooker or baker in the past, so I had a big learning curve ahead of me. I found joy in planning our meals and having the groceries on hand to make them. As you'll soon see, planning what you're going to eat in advance is a surefire success strategy for losing and maintaining weight.

I began a deep dive into recipes and cookbooks. As a vegan, I knew that I ate differently from others, but working through cookbooks opened my eyes to all the healthy food available to me. I kept buying cookbooks. Oy! It seemed as if I owned every single one published!

I started a new weekly regimen of pulling out my cookbooks or recipes from the web and creating a weeklong menu. I filled in a meal planner that my coach had posted on our private Facebook group. I created menus filled with a variety of different vegetables, grains, and legumes. I created different soups. I noted on my meal planner if a recipe came from a cookbook and which page. If a recipe was one I had printed, I attached it to the back of the meal planner itself. I now use my recipe book to hold my meal planner so that it's front and center in the island of my kitchen.

Bite-Sized Nugget

The research is clear: planning your food keeps you on track. Know what you're eating, when you're eating, and how you're going to make good choices.

Call me crazy, but I get a kick out of going into the kitchen in the morning and knowing what I am having for dinner that night. I learned from the reset program how to plan ahead. I began to figure out what meal prep I could do in the morning which made it easier for dinner that night. For example, I could throw some beans into the Instant Pot (an electric pressure cooker) so they would be ready to use at dinner. I could start soaking cashews in the morning that would turn into a creamy soup later.

I am a morning person and I know it's when my energy is highest. Therefore, this is when I did my meal prep. Here's my suggestion: figure out your best time for your meal prep. It might be evenings. If so, find out how to "batch" a few meals so that you're making one and freezing one. I discovered that there are many one-pot meals I could make completely in the morning and heat up for dinner. None of this is rocket science, obviously, but what was changing—besides the way I was planning meals—was my mindset. I was enjoying cooking for the first time ever. Grocery shopping could be quick and focused with an itemized list. Going to the store three or four days out ensured everything stayed fresh.

Most surprising of all from a woman who has always loved eating in restaurants, I was discovering my food tasted better and was healthier! Who knew? When Kevin and I would dine out, I would look at the menu and scoff. "Ha! I could make this better and for a fraction of the cost!" Clearly, my attitude was changing, and as a result I was living my celery test every day and was losing weight.

Bite-Sized Nugget
Figure out your best energy zone; this is your magic time for planning and organizing your eating week.

IN A NUTSHELL

1. It doesn't matter if you've failed before. Ha! If everybody succeeded at diets the first time around, there wouldn't be a multimillion-dollar industry for weight-loss books.
2. Plan for success. Give yourself the celery test to ensure that your actions are consistent with your goals.
3. Create measurable and specific goals. Designate a way to track your progress. Rope in a friend so that you and she are in it together. Remember this quote by James Clear: "When making plans, think big. When making progress, think small."
4. Focus on the success. I will always look back upon my "failing" to reach my goal as a turning point. If I had celebrated my success with the rest of the team, perhaps then I would have continued on a downhill path vs. the rocky roller coaster road I chose.

CHAPTER 13

From Soup to Nuts

All of the A+ Habits
for a B+ Lifestyle

"I always believed if you take care of your body, it will take care of you." —Ted Lindsay

In her book *From Fat to Thin Thinking*, Rita Black discusses becoming a Weight Loss Master. To me, this honorary title means creating daily habits which support your goals every single day. Mastery means you follow these steps in the worst of times (like when my daughter was in ICU for 31 days on life support) or in the best of times (like when I vacationed in Ireland for a month and lost 9.5 pounds and broke the 200-pound mark). Mastering your weight means mastering your day, one day at a time.

The B+ Diet

1. Tons of water daily: I have always known how important drinking water daily is for our health. However, I don't like water. Why would someone pay for a bottle of water which you can get for free from your own tap? Or, as I once heard it said, paying for water is like paying for gravity. My daily diet soda habit for many years was 100–200 ounces (that's over a gallon of diet soda). Today, I have been diet soda–free for over 13 years and counting! In short, my first mindset shift was being open to "learning" to drink water. And yes, it is a skill, a habit we can teach ourselves. Everyone has heard we need to drink half of our body weight in ounces. When I looked at that number and what I weighed at the time, it meant over 150 ounces. Yikes! Needless to say, that goal seemed impossible. As an alternative, I set a goal of 64 ounces daily. It took me several weeks of conscious effort, but now drinking this way is almost automatic. And then I challenged myself to boost my water goal to 80 ounces daily. Another couple of weeks, and voilà, I was doing that. My next goal was 100 ounces, and I got there in just a week. Now, without even thinking about it, I average 150 ounces a day effortlessly. My "liquid habit" includes plain water, herbal tea, and yes, fizzy water. It is now a habit, learned over time and part of my normal day.

Bite-Sized Nugget
Drink your water! And, when you think you've had enough, have a little more.

I realized how much my mindset has shifted since embracing the water habit. Recently, I was at lunch with a friend, and when I left and went to open my car door, I still had my water glass in my hand! It has become so automatic to be holding a glass of water that I walked out with it!

2. Go crazy for veggies: When you are a volume eater like me, it is very comforting to know there is an entire category of food you can eat as much of as you like and not worry about gaining weight. I love veggies—almost all of them.

So many people say they "hate vegetables," and my first thought is their moms might not have cooked them right while they were growing up. My mom cooked green beans so long they were a soggy, limp mess. That was the Southern way she had learned to cook them. Or veggie-haters might not have been exposed to a good variety of veggies growing up. I often counter these claims by sharing that there are thousands to choose from and endless ways to cook them. Start with the ones you like and go from there. Try new ones. Experiment with ways of cooking them—steaming, roasting, air frying, sautéing, and adding them to other things. I add veggies to almost every morning breakfast shake!

There are so many good reasons to eat your veggies daily. Not only are you boosting your health and reducing your risk of heart disease, but it's virtually impossible to overindulge! It's also your secret weapon to avoid getting hungry. Plus, you set a great example to the next generation because you can't overeat veggies—the more you eat, the more weight you lose. Veggies are a great choice to fill up on to keep you from getting hungry, and they are totally guilt-free. You become a great example to your kids, so they don't grow up hating veggies. A great chef I know taught his children this: if you are not hungry enough to eat a carrot, you are not really hungry. You just want to eat.

Bite-Sized Nugget
As your mom always said, "Eat your veggies!"

3. Three meals a day: In today's world where skipping breakfast is touted as a great weight-loss tool, I'm going against the grain and recommending three solid meals a day. Really! I believe knowing you'll be eating breakfast, lunch, and dinner translates into no reason to eat a fourth meal. Of course, the bigger reason is it discourages snacking.

Many folks snack when it has nothing to do with hunger. Instead, they are thirsty. (See another benefit for drinking so much water?) Or they snack because it's become a habit to have popcorn at the movies or watch TV and eat ice cream. The goal with the B+ Diet is to become cognizant of our unhealthy habits and break them.

In his book, *Eat to Live,* Dr. Joel Fuhrman talks about snacking:

"Spending more time in the non-fed state activates biological processes that help to prevent cancer and promote longevity. When the body is not digesting food, it is most effectively detoxifying and healing. If we eat too often, we miss out on these beneficial processes. Snacking is typically recreational eating, and that means excess calories you did not need."

Bite-Sized Nugget

Snacking is not the path to weight loss. It's "dinner and done!"

Tips for sticking to three meals a day:

- After dinner, it is time to "close the kitchen." Some of my clients find success with picking a time and sticking to it. Example: the kitchen closes at 7:00 p.m.
- Right after dinner, brush your teeth as a reminder you are finished eating for the day.
- Remember that food eaten late in the evening often just "sits there" and shows up on the scale in the morning.
- Make sure you eat enough at dinner to ensure you are not hungry later. Eating lots of veggies ensures you stay full.
- Make a big cup of your favorite herbal tea so you have something to hold onto.
- Keep in mind, it is even OK to go to bed a little hungry. It will make your breakfast that much better! You won't die of hunger–and I promise you that you'll live until the morning!

4. Prepping for success: meal planning: Many poor eating choices are due to a lack of planning. You know the drill: you're hungry for dinner and you can't find something easy, healthy, and satisfying. And that's when you decide to have a pizza, order fast food, or order Uber Eats. Big mistake!

Meal planning might seem like a bit more effort up front, but the dividends pay off with both your weight loss and your pocket-book. Why? Because veggies are cheaper than junk food and you can plan your meals based on what's in season and on sale.

Having a routine also aids in turning your weight loss into a habit. For example, every morning for breakfast, I have a protein shake. I never have to think about what I am going to have when I get up. It's always my shake whirled with a little plant milk and veggies. Easy and done!

I also use my breakfast time to plan what I'm having for dinner. It's the perfect time for me, as I'm a morning person. So, while drinking my shake, I'm prepping the veggies for dinner.

Sometimes, if dinner is a one-pot meal (veggie chili or split pea soup), I make it in the morning. Then, that evening all I have to do is heat it up. That little bit of extra work in the morning translates into a hassle-free and healthy meal for dinner. Further, my planning leaves no opening for a poor decision. In short, I've planned my daily food starting at 6 a.m.!

Bite-Sized Nugget
Not planning your meals is planning for failure.

Shopping lists are also a magic ingredient in your weight-loss journey. Working with a list helps prevent impulse purchases (not weight-loss foods) from jumping into your cart. You can turbocharge your shopping list by creating a master list of all your frequently purchased essentials (beans, vinegar, tofu, etc.). Then print it and have it handy, adding other items as needed. As I run out of something, I put a check next to it on the already printed list. At the bottom, there are spaces to write in things not on the list. For example, new things I want to try or need for recipes, like spices or ingredients I don't normally have on hand. Since I buy mostly the same things each time I shop, I can be in and out quickly and know exactly where everything is located.

I also keep a note pad on the front of my fridge to jot down things I need in the kitchen when my preprinted shopping list is not right there.

5. Every bite counts: Whether you are working your way toward your goal weight or maintaining a healthy weight, every bite matters when it comes to the extras! Are you pouring salad dressing over your salad or just dipping the tines of your fork into it?? One of my clients recently shared a photo of her empty salad bowl after lunch. She was so proud, as the bowl was empty instead of swimming with extra dressing on the bottom. I like to use flavored balsamic for my salads. I used to pour it on, and at the end would drink the leftover dressing from the bowl. Did I just admit that? Now I measure just 1 tablespoon, and I've discovered that is plenty. There's none left over, and my expensive balsamic now lasts three times longer!

Bite-Sized Nugget

Tracking is essential to seeing what's working and what's not.

An ounce of nuts or a handful of nuts? One ounce = 157 calories, while 1 cup is a whopping 754 calories! One tablespoon of peanut butter = 95 calories, while just ¼ cup nearly quadruples that to 379 calories.

You get the picture. Keeping track of the small extras determines either success or failure in reaching your goal.

6. Progress, not perfection: The B+ Diet is not about perfection—no one is perfect. It is about making choices in alignment with your goals. If you make a choice to eat a food which is not part of your weight-loss plan, own the choice, track it, and move on. We want to eliminate a diet mentality. We don't make up for a poor choice by skipping the next meal. We make the next meal on plan. Tracking what we eat is how we stay out of denial. If you bite it, you write it. It is about designing a lifestyle and way of eating which allows us to maintain our healthy weight—forever. Part of the process is understanding this one fact.

We cannot eat the way we used to eat, which made us overweight, and ever weigh what we want to weigh. We must make lifetime changes in what we eat, when we eat, and how we think about food if we want lasting changes.

Permanent change begins with being open to doing things in a new way: learning that travel, vacations, holidays, or celebrations don't have to mean giving up on our goals and gaining weight. As we create new B+ habits, we realize our past actions do not determine our future. Our future is dependent on the decisions we are making right now, today, and not what we always did before.

We are creating a new mindset around healthy living and not always being on a diet. And all changes begin with one decision to do something differently—then doing it again and again until it becomes a new habit. And I can tell you without reservation, the longer you do it, the easier it becomes. You have to decide YOU are worth investing the time and energy into you. Is it easy? Heck no! Is it always fun? Of course not! Small consistent daily changes in behavior and choices lead to staggering long-term results. One day, one decision at a time. You are worth it!

7. Limit the "failing foods": Although on this plan there are no "bad" foods, there are poorer choices. I recommend limiting your sweets, alcohol, refined carbs, processed foods, and foods without nutritional value. It doesn't mean that you'll never drink again or indulge in a dish of ice cream; it means that while in the aggressive phases of losing weight, you limit or avoid them.

For example, last fall in Ireland, my husband and I took a tour of the Jameson whiskey distillery. At the end of the tour, we were given one ounce of whiskey. I gave half to my husband and savored every sip of my half. I tracked it, ate normally the rest of the day, and felt no guilt. Each moment we have a choice and make more of them which support our goal creates our success.

And I did the same thing the following year in Scotland.

And I am sure this fall in Scotland, I'll also have a taste of Scotch whisky.

8. The power of protein: As a vegan, I often hear, "Where do you get your protein?" My answer is beans, tempeh, and tofu.

Another form of the same question is "How do you get enough protein?" My fun answer is the same way elephants, rhinos, hippos, bison, wildebeest, horses, manatees and other large animals get theirs: By eating vegetables! These are some of the largest animals on the planet, and they do just fine eating vegetables.

Bite-Sized Nugget
Don't eat foods at odds with your goals.

Another protein myth floating about is that you need to have complete proteins by combining certain foods (e.g., beans with rice). This theory was debunked several years ago. Eating a good variety of plant-based foods daily ensures you have plenty of protein.

Often new vegetarians or vegans are concerned with eating tofu; my answer is that everyone must make their own decision. I choose non-GMO organic tofu and love it. I look at the very healthy Asian cultures which have used tofu as one of their staples for thousands of years. If it works for them, it's working for me!

The B+ Diet philosophy works for everyone: herbivores, carnivores, pescatarians, lacto-ovo vegetarians, and flexitarians.

9. Becoming a clean vegan: At my all-time (recorded) high weight of **350+** pounds, I had been vegan for many years. When you think about it, Oreos, potato chips, and french fries are all vegan. What they are not is healthy.

I first heard the term clean vs. dirty vegan at a San Diego restaurant. I asked the server what was good, and he responded by asking if I was a clean or dirty vegan. He said a dirty vegan was someone who lived on chips and french fries and had never heard of kale.

For a long-term commitment to reaching and maintaining our ideal healthy weight, we must choose clean eating.

10. Make eating healthy a habit—a day in my life: One of my tips for success is to make eating healthy simple and easy. Find foods you like and get into a "good rut." This type of habit eliminates stress and the constant wondering about what you'll eat. When you have your "go to" meals, it is easy to have what you need on hand and to put it together.

For me:

Breakfast is always a protein shake, the healthiest meal of the day.

Lunch is normally a huge salad topped with beans. I vary the veggies and the types of beans. My dressing choice is always a fabulous flavored balsamic vinegar. I have a lot of flavors to choose from. If you haven't searched balsamic vinegars, now is your chance.

Dinner is the meal I vary the most. It's a combination of beans and greens. Veggie soup, veggie chili, and stir-fry meals are a staple of my diet.

I typically don't snack—really! My meals are so filling I don't feel the need and I am not hungry. Remember, if you don't want a carrot, you are not hungry. However, if you are a snacker, limit it to one time a day and make it a healthy snack like veggies. Most importantly, before you snack, ask yourself if you're really hungry. If yes, go ahead and have that snack. If not, rethink the food you've eaten so far in your day. Perhaps you need to add more veggies to your meal. Or maybe your mind is saying hungry while you're actually thirsty. Try having a glass of water first. If you want to snack and aren't actually hungry, this is an opportunity to learn to make another choice. Eating from habit at a certain time of day is one of those mindset shifts we can make to support us in reaching our ideal, healthy weight!

The B+ Diet

A+ Vegetables—

Unlimited; eat at every meal, including breakfast! Please note that "starchy vegetables" including potatoes, corn, winter squash, pumpkins, yams, etc. are limited and can be found under C foods for Carbohydrates. Avocadoes are limited and can be found under Flavor Enhancers.

- Artichoke/hearts
- Asparagus
- Beets
- Brussels sprouts
- Broccoli
- Cabbage
- Carrots
- Cauliflower
- Celery
- Cucumbers
- Eggplant
- Green beans
- Jicama
- Leafy greens (e.g., collard, kale, mustard, turnip, bok choy, kohlrabi)
- Leeks
- Mushrooms
- Okra
- Onions

- Peppers
- Radishes
- Snap peas
- Spaghetti squash
- Sprouts
- Summer squash
- Tomatoes
- Turnips
- Water chestnuts
- Zucchini

B+ Fruits—Good for you, but don't overindulge; 2–3 servings daily.

- Acai
- Ackee
- Apples
- Apricots
- Bananas
- Bilberries
- Blackberries
- Blueberries
- Boysenberries
- Bread fruit
- Cantaloupes
- Cherimoya
- Cherries
- Cranberries

- Currants
- Dates
- Durian
- Elderberries
- Figs
- Gooseberries
- Grapefruit
- Grapes
- Guava
- Honeydew melons
- Huckleberries
- Kiwis
- Kumquat
- Lemons
- Limes
- Lychees
- Mangos
- Mangosteen
- Mulberries
- Muskmelon
- Nectarines
- Oranges
- Papaya
- Passion fruit
- Peaches
- Pears
- Peppers

- Persimmon
- Pineapple
- Plums
- Pluot
- Pomegranate
- Prickly Pear
- Quince
- Raspberries
- Rose Apple
- Starfruit
- Strawberries
- Tamarind
- Tangelo
- Tangerines
- Ugli fruit
- Watermelons
- Xigua melon
- Yellow watermelon

C Foods = Carbohydrates and starchy vegetables. These are fiber-rich foods; Limit to 1-2 servings daily. Always opt for whole grain.

- Barley
- Bread
- Cereal
- Oats
- Pasta
- Pita bread
- Popcorn
- Quinoa
- Tortilla
- Corn
- Potato
- Squash – all other winter types
- Sweet potato
- Yams

Protein—eat at every meal.

- Tofu
- Tempeh
- Beans (soybean, edamame, pinto, etc.)
- Veggie burgers
- Protein powders
- Seitan

Flavor Enhancers: These are the "extras" that add pizzazz to your food! Choose one to two servings per meal using these enhancers sparingly. I recommend that you pull out your measuring spoons and try to use 1 teaspoon at a time.

- Olive Oil
- Condiments
- Nuts
- Seeds
- Salad dressing
- Vegan cheese
- Sauces
- Syrups
- Olives
- Avocado
- Peanut butter and nut butters

"F" Foods—Failing foods that do not support your goals and weight loss.

- Chips
- Chocolate
- Alcohol
- Ice cream
- Fried foods
- Sweetened beverages
- AKA junk foods with lots of empty calories and little nutritional value

IN A NUTSHELL

1. Creating health and reaching our ideal healthy weight is a lifetime commitment. It is not about going on a diet, losing weight, going off the diet, and then ending up heavier than when we started. I know—I have done that countless times. At one point I lost 150 pounds. I found them all again and 50 of their friends. It is about shifting your mindset to change your weight.

2. We can NEVER eat the way we used to eat which made us overweight and ever weigh what we want to weigh. We have to make lifetime changes in what we eat, when we eat, and how we think about food if we want lasting changes.

3. Permanent change begins with being open to doing things in a new way: learning that travel, vacations, holidays, or celebrations don't have to mean giving up on our goals and gaining weight. As we create new B+ habits, we realize our past actions do not determine our future. Our future is dependent on the decisions we are making right now, today, and not what we always did before.

CHAPTER 14

The Bitter Pill to Swallow

Weighing Yourself Daily

"In God we trust. All others must bring data."
—W. Edwards Deming

Facing the Scales

Did someone just say "Get on the scale"? Let's talk about a love-hate relationship!

There have been times in my adult life when I might have gone a year or even longer without weighing myself. Why? Because I was afraid to see the number on the scale. Out of fear, avoidance, or guilt, I just plain didn't want to know what that digital data was saying. I was avoiding the truth. If I hopped on that scale, I would have had to admit that I was obese.

Bite-Sized Nugget
Avoiding the scale is simply avoiding facing the result of your choices.

How many times have you had a binge and decided not to weigh yourself the next day out of fear of what it would say? You decide to wait a few days to "get over" whatever the splurge or poor choices were. And then, because you did not face the scale, the next day you make a few more poor choices and again avoid the scale. Do you see how you just succumbed to a vicious cycle? Here's a different option: What if you *did* get on the scale the next day? What might you see?

- That the gain was not as bad as you thought; you breathe a sigh of relief and get right back on track.
- That you did gain a little weight; you face the consequences and go right back to making great choices today.
- That you learned from the choices you made and go forward armed with new information.

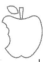

Bite-Sized Nugget
You either lose or you learn.

All the above options are better than putting your head in the sand and ignoring the results of your choices. Avoidance starts the vicious cycle of your weight spiraling out of control. In this program, the B+ Diet, we weigh ourselves daily—no excuses!

It's Just Data

Weighing ourselves daily is a tool; it provides data. Our weight doesn't define us. You are not the number on the scale. What you weigh is statistical data and doesn't make you a good or bad person. It is just information.

Many of us have let the scale determine what our day will look like. Do any of these thoughts sound familiar?

- "I followed my plan to the T yesterday and did not lose weight. I should have eaten the cookie yesterday. What does it matter?"
- "I stayed the same even though I had the cookie yesterday. Guess I will have three of them today."
- "It's not fair. I passed up X and still did not lose weight."

Bite-Sized Nugget
The number on the scale doesn't define you; it's just data.

You Can't Control the Scale

When you are setting goals, base them on achievements over which you have 100 percent control. You don't have control over the number on the scale. Yes, I just wrote that. You have control over your eating choices and staying true to your commitment. However, you often can't control the scale. Our bodies experience natural ups and down for a variety of reasons, including water retention, medications, muscle soreness, time of the month, hormones, sleep, and inflammation. The results of our choices—good or bad—often don't show up for days. What you weigh today is not always a direct reflection of what you ate yesterday.

Base your successes on meeting actionable and measurable goals like the following:

- Drinking X ounces of water
- Exercising for X number of minutes
- Following the eating plan without variation for 48 hours
- Choosing not to consume sugar, caffeine, chocolate, etc., for 24 hours

All the points above are choices that you have control over. Making friends with your scale can be a turning point in your journey to reach and maintain your healthy weight for life. When surveyed, people who lost weight and have maintained that loss for over five years often cite weighing themselves regularly as a key to their success. By being aware of their daily weight, they notice quickly if their weight is going up and can choose to act immediately.

During my first fifteen years of coaching, I recommended weighing weekly. My belief was that the daily fluctuations would be too discouraging to someone following a plan. Dieters might give up. There is a saying I remember which goes something like this: "Just because you believe something doesn't make it true." I've changed my belief. When I had the opportunity to participate in a test group about the mindset of eating, I was eager to participate. And because I am a coach, I made a commitment to myself to be coachable to learn new tools.

One of the guidelines was weighing myself daily. This was something I had never done. When I was in Weight Watchers so many times, I never weighed in except weekly and only at my meetings. In fact, weighing daily is a key differentiating factor of this diet versus Optifast, Jenny Craig, Nutrisystem, and Weight Watchers. I adopted weighing in daily and created a log the very first day. The first month was very eye opening as I watched those numbers daily.

Given the thousands of pounds I have lost and found, I know that I lose weight more slowly than many people. I stayed exactly on my plan, and yet sometimes the scale went up. Other days, it went down. There didn't seem to be any rhyme or reason since I was eating much the same day after day. However, at the end of the month, I was down 10 pounds. My key learning was that even with the ups and downs, I was trending down.

I've noticed patterns in my weight loss over the past year. This knowledge has given me freedom from emotional attachment to the numbers on the scale. And what I found interesting writing this chapter is that prior to today, I had seven weight-loss days in a row, which is highly unusual for me. To be honest, the weight loss was freaking me out a bit. Upon weighing myself today, I remained exactly the same, which was oddly comforting. My mindset has made a 180-degree turn, and I now advise all my coaching clients to weigh themselves daily.

Seven Rules for Success

Making friends with your scale turns it into a powerful tool for success instead of your enemy. Following are my weighing rules:

1. Make weighing-in a daily habit—I have an old-fashioned balance beam scale (the ones that are in a doctor's office with weights which you move along the top). Its top advantage is consistency; it stays at the same number no matter how many times you get off and on. However, I also recently bought an Aria scale. It's the high-tech answer to weight loss in that it has an app, syncs with your phone, and creates solid graphs and visual aids. Whichever scale you choose, pick one and weigh yourself religiously every day. The charts and graphs will also provide motivation as you see the numbers decline.

2. Learn from the data—When you learn your specific patterns, you are able to release 99 percent of your emotional attachment to the number. Obviously, I get excited when I release weight and am a bit disappointed when I am up a bit. However, the numbers don't throw me off track, and I think back to the day before to glean anything helpful. For example, this year I have fallen in love with pho—a fabulous Vietnamese soup. I'm on a quest to find the best pho in the world and am even working on creating my own perfect recipe. The last time I had this Vietnamese delicacy, I was up a startling 1.5 pounds the next morning! Hmmm. I deduced that the soup must have had a ton of salt and I was therefore suffering from water retention. The tiny weight gain did not take me off track, and I upped my water intake over the next few days. Three days later, those 1.5 pounds were gone.

3. Remember the scale is just a number—Your value is not measured on a scale. I have gone from calling my scale "The Metal Monster" when my weight was up to my "Happy Hardware" when I was losing weight. It is just a number, and those numbers vary from day to day. Keep your commitment to yourself daily, stay the course, and remain persistent.

4. Know fluctuations are normal—Trends are what matter. You need the daily numbers to determine your personal weight-loss patterns. As mentioned, these ups and down have many causes, but keep your focus on the big picture.

5. Weigh yourself at the same time—In addition to weighing daily, weigh yourself at approximately the same time every day. The best time is the first thing in the morning after using the bathroom and before you eat or drink anything. One glass of water can up the scale by half a pound!

6. Never avoid the scale—Face it and own it. Even if the news is bad, it's temporary, and action can be taken immediately. Getting on the scale even when you think you have gained weight is called taking responsibility for your choices.

7. Travel with your scale—Did I scare you yet? While your first reaction may be "What?," I have found it pays amazing dividends. Vacation doesn't mean you abandon your healthy living goals. On a recent trip to Ireland for one month, we packed my scale and I weighed and tracked my weight every single day. While it may be a bit different reading than my scale at home, it does show daily ups and downs. Being aware of making smart choices when you are away from home creates habits which last a lifetime.

Making a vacation about memories instead of food is a mindset shift. Believe me when I say you can have as much fun and come home feeling good about yourself. It's OK to try some of the local foods, but don't make it your focus. You will be rewarded when you step on the scale after returning home.

IN A NUTSHELL

1. Don't avoid the scale. It's merely data that lets you make better decisions. Weigh yourself daily so that, if necessary, you can quickly correct your eating.
2. You are not what you weigh. Make sure to set goals that you control.
3. Track your weight. Whether you chart your journey on an app or in an Excel spreadsheet, it's a great visual tool for seeing your progress.

CHAPTER 15

On a Silver Platter

Tracking Your Journey

"Data will talk to you if you're willing to listen." —Jim Bergeson

The Power of Data

Similar to me recommending that you weigh yourself daily, I encourage, pressure, proselytize, and demand that you create a food and exercise diary. It is data; you need data to move down the scale.

I keep both trackers to see at a glance how I'm doing. For my exercise, for example, I use the tennis shoe available as a bonus at www.TheBPlusDiet.com/Bonus. Note that it is a 100-day tracker. For every workout, I color in the shoe (I love my colored markers), thereby reinforcing my positive actions.

The research is overwhelmingly strong that a food diary is your secret weapon to getting and keeping the weight off. A study from the Kaiser Permanente Center for Health Research has shown that people who keep a food diary lose twice as much weight as those who don't. According to the lead author of the study, "The more food records people kept, the more weight they lost." Are you convinced yet?

Setting Goals

Since we are committed to tracking, your essential first steps are to weigh yourself, take your measurements, and commit to actionable and specific goals. Set a goal weight and write it down. If you're not sure what your weight should be, feel free to consult the Centers for Disease Control or the American Cancer Society for a simple weight chart based upon your height.

Most of us know that goals must be specific. They should also be measurable, attainable, relevant, and time-bound: SMART.

Amorphous Goal	Specific Goal
I will exercise more often.	I am committed to walking Mondays, Tuesdays, and Wednesdays at 8 a.m.
I will eat more vegetables.	I will have 8 or more servings of non-starchy veggies daily.

Amorphous Goal	Specific Goal
I will lose 50 pounds by my wedding.	I will follow the program religiously, track my food intake, and write down my exercise daily.
I will limit my starch servings.	I will have two or fewer starch servings daily.
I will reduce the amount of caffeine.	Each day I will have two ounces less than the day before.
I will start drinking more water.	I will drink 80 ounces or more daily.
I will eat dinner earlier.	My dinner will be done by 8 p.m.
I will cut down my wine drinking.	I will have no more than one glass of wine weekly.

Are you surprised that I put "lose 50 pounds by my wedding" as an amorphous goal? I did that because what I've learned from gaining and losing over 2,500 pounds in my lifetime is that your body determines how much weight it will release at its own pace. You cannot control whether you will lose two pounds or four pounds this week, but you *can* control that you will do everything in your power to make it possible and not sabotage the effort. I did lose an average of two pounds per week, but I also had weeks where I lost zero weight or gained weight! During those troublesome weeks, I reviewed my food diary and noticed that sodium was a major culprit. If I had pho for lunch, I knew my weight would go up for the next two days before it settled back down.

Bite-Sized Nugget

As part of your tracking, make sure to take a picture of yourself on the first day of every month. It's your visual narrative of your weight-loss journey.

Short-Term Goals for Long-Term Success

If you know you want to get down to a size 6 and you're currently a size 22, your goal seems daunting. Heck, I was a size 5X with a goal to get to a size 4. I did it, but I also took baby steps and created bite-sized goals. One of my motivating mini goals was to find an outfit which was a bit too small. I hung it on my bedroom door where I saw it daily. I tried it on once a week until it fit. When it fit, I picked another one and did the same thing. I knew that it would take me at least one full year, if not longer, to reach my goal. My mental headspace was geared up for the long haul.

Dr. Edward Banfield of Harvard University took a deep dive into why certain people achieved great success and others didn't. His main conclusion? Long-term perspective. Successful people are long-term thinkers who reverse engineer their goals, so they know exactly what to do to achieve them. Read Brian Tracy's perspective on this.

The Pen Is Mightier Than the Keyboard

Of course, I know that there are apps to track your weight, food, water, and sleep. However, I encourage you and all of my clients to adopt the pen. Handwriting activates parts of your brain used in memory and recall. Further, writing by hand allows you to think more thoroughly about the information you're recording. Knowing that you must track four glasses of wine might just deter you from pouring an extra glass or two.

Bite-Sized Nugget
Track every morsel you put in your mouth in real time using a pen or pencil.

If you're reading this and ready to exclaim, "But tracking is tedious, boring, and inconvenient," I have an answer for you: Perhaps. There are work-arounds. I urge you to take a photo on your phone of your meals if you can't record them in real time. Don't be afraid to take your tracker with you for out-of-the-house dining. However, I reassure you that tracking is the proven method for seeing what you're eating, when you're eating, and what choices you're making. A 2019 study published in the journal *Obesity* showed that it took participants only 15 minutes per day to record what they ate and drank.

Tracking Allows for Reviewing and Revising

Every time I start with a new group of weight-loss clients, I'll have one person who is stalled with losing weight yet shouting to the rooftops that she is following the program perfectly. The first question I always ask is this: "Can you send me your food tracker?" If the answer is that there is no tracker, then I know immediately why she isn't succeeding. You can't fix what you can't see.

If, however, my client has a tracker, I'm able to provide an outsider's view and add value immediately. Sometimes I see too many nuts, avocados, or too much olive oil. Other times I note heaping spoonfuls of peanut butter or oversize portions. The bottom line is that the tracker not only works for an outsider but it works for you. When you get stalled, you can easily review your week to determine what choices were good and what were not so good. The power of change and choice is in your hands.

IN A NUTSHELL

1. Visual reminders help keep us on track. It's one of the reasons I encourage you to track your food intake and exercise schedule daily. I also want you to take photos so that you stay motivated; it might seem as if you're not losing weight, but then when you see the evidence, your momentum returns.
2. Divide your goals into baby steps. You are working on a lifelong journey, not a sprint.

CHAPTER 16

No Sugarcoating Here
Why There Are
No Cheat Days

"Cheating is a choice, not a mistake." —Unknown

When you embrace the B+ Diet mindset, you recognize that it's all about choice; it's about choosing what to eat, when to eat, and how it makes you feel. There are no foods that are forbidden. However, if you want to lose weight, you should make better choices. Stay away from the "failing foods" or what we call the "F" foods as compared to the B+ foods. Examples of "F" foods include fried foods, potato chips, ham, and nachos. See chapter 13 for a quick review of the program.

It's Not Cheating, It's a Choice

As a result, there are no cheat days. Cheating implies deviousness, as in cheating on a test, cheating on your taxes, or cheating on your spouse. Yikes!

Eating a cookie is not unethical or immoral. What we eat or don't eat is not a question of morality or ethics; it is simply a choice. There are great choices, good choices, mediocre choices, poor choices, and bad choices. What these options all have in common is the word choice—not cheat.

Bite-Sized Nugget

There are no cheat days, just choice days. Choose the right food to hit your goals.

The Myth of a Food Addiction

When it comes to excuses for not losing the weight, I've heard them all. Heck! I've said them all myself. However, the one phrase that never rings true for me is this one: "I'm a food addict." Really?

Telling yourself that you're a food addict transfers the responsibility of your clean eating habits and heaps them on a disease for which there is no diagnosis. Further, it turns you into a victim. "Oh, I can't lose weight because I have a food addiction." When you release yourself of that victim mentality, you morph into a powerful role whereby you are in control. Say to yourself instead: "I choose the wrong foods often. Now, I'm on a path to making better choices."

Old Phrases	New Phrases that Put You in Control
I have a food addiction.	I choose the wrong foods often. Now, I'm on a path to making better choices.
Today is my cheat day.	There are no cheat days; every day I make good choices.
I need my comfort food.	Food is fuel, not comfort.
I love my treats.	Treats are for dogs, and I'm not a dog. I treat myself to indulgences, like a mani-pedi, bubble bath, etc.
I goofed this morning so I'm giving up on the whole day.	No goofs; I'm either losing or learning.
I'm never going to have ice cream again in my life; it's a bad food.	Food is merely food; I'll simply delay it today, not deny it forever.

Quitting Habits that No Longer Serve Our Goals

My love affair with diet soda began 14 years ago. Pouring a Diet Coke into an iced glass was my version of a treat. Again, that was 220 pounds ago. Today, I know that I can still drink a can of soda whenever I want. But today, I choose not to drink it.

Labeling a food off-limits forever is a mistake. It means that we are on a diet and then will be off a diet. Instead, a lifestyle decision means making better choices. Delay, not deny.

Bite-Sized Nugget
Don't tell yourself that there are forbidden foods; it will only make you crave them more. Instead: it's delay, not deny.

Dinner and Done

One of the keys to weight-loss success is the mantra "dinner and done." In short, it means the mouth and kitchen are closed for the evening. Similar to the power of starting the day with a healthy breakfast, the end of the day concludes with a healthy dinner.

I recommend eating dinner before 8 p.m., but it's not a hard-and-fast rule. I'd still rather you eat a healthy late dinner than no dinner at all. Note that studies are clear that when food is consumed late at night, your body is more likely to store those calories as fat and gain weight rather than burn it as energy.

Dinner and done also prevents you from snacking or even thinking about it. There's no popcorn, nuts, or fruit. Good night! Here are suggested behaviors that signal you are done for the evening:

- Brush your teeth
- Start the dishwasher
- Turn off kitchen lights
- Get into your pj's
- Finish your tracker and review and/or send to your coach.

Divorcing Behaviors from Old Habits

Pretend that every time you went to the movies, you bought yourself a giant tub of hot buttered popcorn. Yum! Now, however, you are on a mission to make better choices, beginning with delaying having popcorn until you feel it's the perfect time. So, let me ask you: Will going to the movies support your new goal? Probably not. You've developed a habit as well as a connection: movies = popcorn. Other folks only smoke when they're drinking; their connection is: alcohol = smoking. Research shows that divorcing these actions from each other equals success. It's one of the reasons that smokers give up their habit more successfully when they are on vacation, because they've disassociated the habits from their environment.

The flip side of unlinking behaviors to get rid of bad habits is that you can link two behaviors to form good habits. For example, if you'd like to keep a promise to work out four days per week, tie it to another habit like quitting work at 5 p.m. Closing down your computer = time to work out.

Researcher Peter Gollwitzer calls the marrying of two behaviors action triggers. One study analyzed people's success in accomplishing easy or hard goals. With easy goals, the use of action triggers increased success from 78% to 84%. However, with hard goals, action triggers nearly tripled the chance of success; goal completion went up from 22% to a jaw-dropping 62%!

Going back to our movie example, you can create a new trigger so that when you walk in and smell the popcorn, you immediately buy a bottle of water (or bring your own). Or, if that action requires too much self-control, for the time being, watch your movies at home. You are switching the environment and divorcing the two activities from each other to boost your chances of success.

Old Habit	New Habit
I never eat breakfast.	I eat breakfast within an hour of getting out of bed.
I always eat popcorn at the movies.	I take a bottle of water to the movies.
I always have pizza on Friday.	I find a new recipe every Friday.
I eat whatever and whenever I want.	I track every bite that goes in my mouth.
I sauté my food with olive oil.	I sauté my food with veggie broth.
I'm afraid to get on the scale.	I weigh myself daily.
I wear baggy clothes to hide my body.	I wear form-fitted clothes to feel good about myself.

Old Habit	New Habit
If I eat one bite, I'll eat the whole thing.	If I choose one bite, I can stop.
I am starving.	I can wait until the next meal to eat and will be fine.

IN A NUTSHELL

1. The language of food is rife with emotion: falling off the wagon (what wagon?), cheat days, treat days, and comfort food. Food is merely fuel; make the right choices to hit your goals.
2. A lifestyle means that no foods are forbidden. Simply tell yourself that it might not be today, but it will be some day.
3. Breaking and starting new habits is hard. Set yourself up for success by seeing if you can create action triggers that keep you on the right path or change the environment to change the habit.

Chapter 17

Travel Is the Spice of Life

How to Travel Without Losing Your Way

"Travel is the only thing you buy that makes you richer."
—Anonymous

Excuses Make the World Go Round

Travel. It's the food and the fun, right? Not really. Coming home from a vacation heavier than when you departed doesn't sound like fun to me! I know how hard it is to get every ounce off.

So, I travel, but I put in the work to make sure I stay on track. Trust me, I've heard every excuse in the book when it comes to eating and traveling:

- Oh, I'm on vacation. I can eat what I want.
- Food doesn't count on vacation.
- I'm taking a vacation from my food plan.

Joyce Marter, in her book *The Financial Mindset Fix: A Mental Fitness Program for an Abundant Life,* shares how she was stuck writing that very book. Eventually she meets with a Buddhist monk who explains that she needs to "weaken the negative narrative of excuses" and tune in to a positive perspective. When she gave up excuses, she finally finished the book, which is available now.

Now is your time to get past the rationalizations and the excuses. This chapter is focused on what I learned during the past three years to make travel and weight loss work.

The most important factor to understand about traveling is that you must pack your mindset first; you must make the commitment that you will do what it takes to enjoy new sights, sounds, cultures, and yes, a few new foods. Taste it or try it, but you don't have to eat the whole thing.

On my first trip to Ireland, for example, I tried Guinness. On my second stop at a pub, I drank water. After all, I had already tasted the beer and I knew what it tasted like! On our trip to Costa Rica, I told myself that if a dessert sounded outrageously delicious, I would order it. If, after one bite, it didn't score a 10 (on a 10-point scale), I wouldn't have another bite. If it really was a 10, then I would have three bites. Three bites let you truly enjoy. It's also the beginning of practicing control and kicking to the curb the "clean your plate club."

Bite-Sized Nugget

If you're committed to success, there's always an answer; if you're not committed to your success, there's always an excuse.

Set a Goal for Your Trip

Before you travel, set a goal for the time period you will be gone. Choose a realistic and achievable goal which is doable and motivates you to stay the course. You might choose that your goal is to maintain your weight for your trip. My goal for 30 days in Ireland was to release 5 or more pounds—an average of 1.25 pounds each week. In addition, I also had a stretch goal, which was to lose over 9 pounds. A stretch goal is something which can seem a bit of a reach in the time available and yet is amazing to shoot for—a stretch! And I did lose 9.5 pounds, breaking the 200-pound mark in Ireland!!

With these tips, you will see how doable it was for me to release 9.5 pounds during my vacation and come home feeling proud of my choices. Most importantly, I felt strong and powerful with the knowledge that not only could I stick to my plan, but that I did it! And you can too.

Remember how I shared about staying motivated by creating mini goals? For this trip, I set two pairs of jeans by the door. I wanted to pack them, but they were just too tight. Can you imagine my elation upon coming home and finding out that they fit?

On the Road Again

Road trips are the easiest to master since you have the luxury to take along all the tools and supplies necessary to support your weight-loss journey. It's also easy to stop when necessary and convenient to resupply. I personally tend to "overstock" my car, knowing I have everything I need to eat healthy and feel satisfied. In July of 2019, my husband and I took a two-week road trip to Indianapolis and back for my company convention. Here's a handy checklist:

1. **Big Cooler, aka Your Traveling Fridge:** Your cooler acts as your mobile refrigerator. It's simple to restock as needed, and most hotels even have free ice. Your goal is to fill it with the healthy foods that support your goals.
- Almond milk
- Fresh veggies
- Fresh fruit
- Salad makings
- Condiments
- Prepared Foods—hummus, smoothies, etc.
- Water bottles

2. **Big Box, aka Your Traveling Pantry:** This is your dry foods which don't need to be refrigerated.
- Protein shake
- Dried beans
- Canned beans

- Herbs and spices
- Onions
- Bananas, apples, oranges
- Dried fruits and nuts
- Tea bags
- Stevia

3. **Tools You Can Use:** These are the tools you need to be able to eat on the road; it unchains you from having every meal in a restaurant. I have honed this list down to a science.

- Cutlery—two forks, spoons, and knives
- Two bowls
- Two plates
- Small cutting board and chef's knife
- Teakettle
- Two teacups
- Can opener
- Instant pot (to cook dried beans, which then go into cooler)
- Mini blender
- Two shake containers
- Different size baggies

4. **Travel Scale:** I travel with my scale—*always*. After all, one of the key components of the B+ Diet is weighing yourself daily. How can you remain accountable without a scale? I have a lightweight Renpho Scale which syncs with a program on my computer and tracks my numbers. This one tool is a direct link between my actions and my results.

Up in the Air

Traveling by air obviously limits your options. However, I've created a "kitchen suitcase," which is a mini version of the tools detailed above. For long trips, the only food I pack is my protein powder (individually packaged) plus two shaker cups and my favorite herb tea.

Here are four tips for the flight:

1. **Request a Special Meal from the Airline**—With new travel restrictions, thanks to COVID, food may or may not be an option except in business and first class. If you can request a special meal which supports your goals, select it.

2. **Carry on Packaged TSA-Friendly Foods**—TSA rules change all the time and even from agent to agent. My favorite items to bring on board are protein shake single-serving packets to mix with water on the plane. Other faves include fresh chopped veggies. If you're doing a make-your-own-salad with garbanzo beans, for example, drain the beans and then put in a clear plastic bag. The last time I went through TSA, however, mine were confiscated. Check here for the latest rules: https://www.tsa.gov/travel/security-screening/whatcanibring/food

3. **Buy a Huge Bottle of Water**—Nothing feels worse than being dehydrated and waiting for a flight attendant to serve you a glass of water. I also take my own vessel (32 oz) and fill it before I board.

4. **Take More Than You Need**—Thanks to weather and travel days, bring more food and water than you think you'll

need. Often, there are not even snacks on the plane due to safety concerns.

Eating Along the Road

Here's a hidden gem for eating healthy on the road: Subway! Although it has a lot of unhealthy choices too, I discovered that its chopped veggie salad is a winner.

Here's how I do it. I order the chopped veggie salad and ask for extras of all the veggies; they always say yes. Some of the outlets now offer oregano and other delish salt-free spice blends. I also get an avocado on top, which I mash up to become my salad dressing. I bring in edamame beans and add to my salad. Voilà! A healthy on-the-road meal which is satisfying and filling and very reasonably priced. Not only a great travel option, but it is also my go-to place when out doing errands when home.

Plan Ahead for Restaurant Meals

In this day and age, with so many folks having special dietary needs and allergies, virtually every restaurant has an online menu for you to review to see how its menu fits your plan. Look at menus in new ways with your imagination. Don't just look at the individual menu options but at the ingredients. Can you vary an appetizer to make it your dinner? Can you "steal" the beans from the taco salad to make a healthy Mexican option for yourself? If the restaurant has an ingredient on hand, it can usually make something special for you.

Bite-Sized Nugget

Burger King was right in 1974—have it your way! Don't be embarrassed or intimidated to order what you need to stay on your plan.

We were invited to join a bunch of friends for dinner at Applebee's (a place I would never choose to eat). However, I did want to spend time with our friends. I pored over the menu and saw only two possible choices. I knew I could order a plain salad, and they had broccoli on the menu. When the server took my order, I asked for two side salads, veggies only, and asked for it to be placed on a dinner plate. I also asked for the broccoli to be steamed plain. She informed me it came with butter on it, and I asked to leave the butter off. She said she did not think they could do that, as it came with butter. I very nicely told her I bet they could and asked her to check with the chef. She came back with a somewhat shocked look on her face and said, "We can do that." You just have to ask for what you want. When my dinner came, I added the beans I had in my purse on top of the salad, along with the steamed broccoli and the salad dressing (balsamic vinegar) I had brought with me. None of the other diners noticed or paid attention to what I was ordering or eating. I had a nice time with friends and stayed on my plan.

We often eat many of our meals in the hotel room when traveling. Virtually every breakfast is in our room because we start the day with our shake. I navigate to stores that stock fresh veggies once I arrive in a new city.

Since I can't bring all of my traveling supplies with me on an airplane trip, I rely upon the kindness of the hotel kitchen. Every single hotel I visited was happy to provide silverware, a large salad bowl, and teakettles. Not only did I save a good deal of money eating meals in my room, but I also felt great about what I was eating. Don't be afraid to ask for what you need.

At one hotel in the very small town of Donegal, Ireland, a lovely woman at the front desk was curious as to why we were shopping and asking for a salad bowl. I explained that my hubby and I are plant-based and were having trouble finding meals which fit our plan. She felt so bad that she told us she was going to speak to the hotel chef and see what she could do. It turned out the chef created a special meal just for us (not on the menu), and we had a great dinner that night. It was the only meal we ate in the hotel dining room!

Suggested List of Healthy Travel Options: Always check online before you go.

Fast Food

- *Chipotle:* Bean burritos (black beans), Sofritas bowl (black beans and brown rice), salad with veggies, black beans, hold the dressing and add avocado.
- *El Pollo Loco:* Bean bowl, steamed broccoli, salad greens with chopped veggies, beans and pico de gallo and avocado.

- *McDonald's:* Side salad, hold the dressing, and apple slices.
- *BurgerFi:* Vegan Beyond Burger in a lettuce wrap.
- *Pick Up Stix:* Mandarin Garden Salad, Buddha's Feast. Note: The chain will always sub tofu in any entrée, and always ask for no oil.

Chain Sit-down Restaurants

- *Jason's Deli*: Taco salad with beans (omit cheese and sour cream), fresh fruit bowl, spinach veggie wrap (omit cheese), organic vegetable soup, steamed veggies, fresh fruit bowl without dip, great salad bar, and zucchini grillini (hold the cheese). Build your own veggie sandwich and black bean and corn salad.
- *Cheesecake Factory:* Edamame side and vegan cobb salad.
- *Red Robin:* Vegan burger in a lettuce wrap.
- *Loving Hut:* Vegan chain across the country.
- *Sweetgreen:* Miso Bowl, Shroomami Bowl, curry chickpea bowl, spicy Thai salad, hummus tahini, and lentil and avocado salads.
- *Veggie Grill and Native Foods:* Both are vegan chains growing across the country.
- *True Food Kitchen*: Veggie plate, kale guacamole, ancient grains bowl, butternut squash pizza, tomato and arugula pizza, TLT sandwich.

- *BJ's:* Lentil soup with ancient grains, enlightened vegetarian quinoa bowl, kale and roasted Brussels sprouts salad (hold the cheese).
- *Snappy Salads*: Grilled avocado salad or falafel wrap.
- **Vietnamese restaurants:** All offer veggie pho; just make sure to order veggie broth.
- **Chinese**: Tons of veggies and tofu, and ask for no oil.
- **Whole Foods**: Always lots of great options at their deli, including soups and salad bars. Also, a great place to stock your travel fridge.

There is a great app called Happy Cow (www.happycow.net), which lists vegan restaurants all over the world.

We have talked about road trips in our cars, air travel, and I want to mention one other area. We have a motorhome and love traveling. A lot of the guidelines for road trips still apply, with one big plus. In our motorhome we have our kitchen stocked with all the tools we have at home, including our Vitamix and our Instapot.

When you are committed to losing weight, you can still travel and enjoy life. Plan ahead, take what you need, and be mindful along the way. You always have a choice.

Safe journey and happy, healthy travels.

IN A NUTSHELL

1. Planning is key when traveling. You have to pack and plan your food, but if you're committed, you'll be successful.
2. Do your homework. Seek out veggie-friendly restaurants, review menus in advance, use apps to discover new places.
3. Be kind. You are a guest in a hotel or in a restaurant. Ask graciously, and you'll be surprised at how willing people are to help.

CHAPTER 18

Waking and Shaking Things Up

Adding Healthy Smoothies to Breakfast

"Eating McDonald's after a workout is like taking a shower and putting your dirty underwear back on."
—Anonymous

Ahhhh! Doesn't a shake sound great for breakfast? It does, but it must be a healthy shake/smoothie. So, let's review:

A shake is not dessert
A shake does not include ice cream

A shake doesn't include sugar, fat, or cream

A shake is not a Frappuccino

A shake is not a Dairy Queen Blizzard

So, What is a Healthy Shake?

Instead, a healthy shake includes vegetables, one fruit, and a concentrated protein source. Of course, my fave vegan shake is Café Latte, and you can find more info here: (https://tinyurl.com/BplusDietShake). This is my choice because it is a high-quality, complete meal replacement and nutritional supplement containing nearly 50 *different* superfoods!

My magic formula is cashew milk (25 C per cup), carrots, banana, romaine lettuce (and feel free to mix up the greens), and fennel. Of course, yours can include kale, apple, carrots, plus your protein source. If you don't add a protein powder, I recommend either beans or tofu. Protein is essential. Protein is what provides satiety and keeps us from getting hungry two or three hours later.

And here's my latest little secret: I put the entire banana, including the peel, into my shake! Approximately 35% of the fruit is the peel, and it's often simply discarded, ending up in landfills. By eating it, I get a boost of immunity, fiber, vitamins, and essential amino acids.

Bite-Sized Nugget

There's a difference between a healthy shake and an indul-
gent milkshake.

Turning Your Routine into a Habit

For over 14 years, I have started my day with my healthy shake.
It works for me and it will work for you. Why? Because you
start your day with a healthy wake-up to your metabolism. Further, your healthy start puts you in the right mood, revved up
with a positive attitude that says, "Yes, I can control my hunger
and make healthy choices."

Another reason I adore having the exact same thing every
day is that it eliminates choice. I'll never make a wrong move
at breakfast because I've planned for it (planning ahead is a key
for long-term success) and it's now become a habit. The harsh
reality is this: the more choices you have to make throughout
the day, the harder it becomes to make good ones, including
about what to eat. Less choices = more correct ones.

I plan for my shake daily by making sure I have the proper
ingredients on hand. In fact, every night I put out the dry ingredients for the next day (along with my workout clothes), so I am
ready to kick off the morning on the right path.

Since the entire purpose of this book is to advocate how
healthy eating is a series of lifetime choices, I recommend starting the day with an unfailing morning habit. If you start the

day off properly, you won't fall into the old habit of thinking you've already gone off the rails, so you might as well binge all day. Remember: you are not on a diet, but on a lifelong mission.

Of course, feel free to replace another meal with a healthy shake. One of my clients likes to make a healthy chocolate shake after dinner. It's her way of signifying the end of the day, the end of her eating, and the joy of having a mini dessert.

The Fallacy of Intermittent Fasting

You'll find that many weight-loss coaches recommend that you limit your eating to a few hours per day. For instance, the 16/8 method recommends skipping breakfast and restricting your daily eating period to 8 hours, such as 1–9 p.m. Then you fast for 16 hours in between. Wrong!

My experience, having coached thousands of weight-loss clients, is that it translates into eating the exact same amount of food, but with a heavy dose of misery. Skipping breakfast causes headaches and nervousness; it never allows for your body to fully wake up. Virtually all research studies on fasting are based upon research from animals, and the data on humans is decidedly mixed, with some participants actually gaining weight!

Bite-Sized Nugget
Stop skipping breakfast! It's your secret weapon for starting the day on a healthy note.

I find the story of the hummingbird particularly illuminating. This tiny bird burns food so fast that it eats almost three times its daily weight per day. To sleep during particularly cold temperatures, its body temperature drops almost 50 degrees and its heart rate plummets from 500 beats per minute to fewer than 50. It enters a state of torpor. To fully wake up, these ruby-throated hummingbirds flap their wings ferociously and then start eating to restore their energy and core temperature.

We are like the hummingbirds. To fully wake up, we must both move and eat.

Bottom line, starting your day with a healthy shake keeps you humming right along!!!

Another key question to ask yourself about any eating habit is this: Can you eat like that forever? If you don't see yourself permanently eating only protein or forever fasting for 16 hours a day, then you have a diet and not a lifestyle.

Doing something only to lose weight is a diet mindset. We are talking about creating healthy lifestyle mindsets; not only to lose the weight but also to maintain the weight loss for life.

Bite-Sized Nugget

The B+ Diet is a forever lifestyle choice. If you hear of the Keto diet or intermittent fasting and you can't see yourself doing it for the rest of your life, then you've chosen a long-term failing proposition.

IN A NUTSHELL

1. Eating the same thing for either break-fast, lunch, or dinner eliminates choice and keeps you on a healthy path.
2. A protein shake is a great swap for break-fast as long as you don't overwhelm it with sugar, cream, fat, or too many fruits.
3. Always eat breakfast; it revs up your metab-olism and allows you to face the day with energy and verve.

CHAPTER 19

Full of Beans

Why I Chose to Go Vegan

"Nothing will benefit human health and increase the chances for survival of life on Earth as much as the evolution to a vegetarian diet." —Albert Einstein

I've been a vegan now for 27 years. I decided that a whole-food, plant-based diet was best for me for three reasons: (1) my health, (2) the animals, and (3) the environment.

However, you do not need to give up meat, fish, or chicken on the B+ Diet. You do want to embrace veggies. Throughout this chapter, I'll provide you my reasons for becoming a vegan, and the choice, of course is yours. Don't forget: this book is a judgment-free zone. Make choices which work for you.

Bite-Sized Nugget

You don't have to give up meat to succeed on the B+ Diet. However, lowering your meat consumption will boost your weight loss.

Giving Up Meat Slowly

I remember that I became intrigued about becoming a vegetarian in the 1990s. I was at a realtor conference and the speaker highlighted learnings from *Fit for Life* by Harvey and Marilyn Diamond. I came home and devoured the book. Reading about the inhumane treatment of chickens boiled my blood, so to speak. As a result, both my husband and I gave up poultry.

I took a deeper dive into the plant world when I read *Beyond Beef* by Jeremy Rifkin. At this time, my family loved eating at Burger King. Interestingly enough, the book jacket advised readers to go buy the biggest, juiciest burger they could, because after reading this book, they would never want to eat beef again. He was right—we gave up beef!

Six months later, I decided to continue my vegetarian discovery process. The book which ultimately had the greatest impact on me was *Diet for a New America* by John Robbins. Robbins addressed not only the health issues associated with a meat-eating society, but also explained the cruel processes involved in rearing and slaughtering animals. Note: At the end of this chapter, I've listed my fave books and documentaries to help you decide.

Clean Vegan vs. Dirty Vegan

I've made the distinction between a clean vegan and a dirty vegan because when I first became a vegetarian, I was living the life of the latter. In other words, I was eating onion rings, Cheetos, potato chips, and soda. All of these are vegan, but none of them are good for me or for you. These foods are an example of "failing foods." They don't improve your health. I understand that you might indulge occasionally, but it doesn't mean you have failed: it simply means you've made a choice, and at the next opportunity, you'll choose differently.

Bite-Sized Nugget

If you're going to be vegan, make sure you opt to become a "clean vegan," eating the rainbow of fruits, vegetables, beans, and legumes.

The Life-Saving Benefits of a Whole Food Plant-Based Diet

Finally, the benefits of a vegan diet are being screamed from the rooftops by renowned doctors such as Joel Fuhrman, Michael Greger, Alona Pulde, Caldwell Esselstyn and T. Colin Campbell. The essence of all these authors' research is that a plant-based diet can reverse and prevent disease.

In the landmark book, *The China Study: The Most Comprehensive Study of Nutrition Ever Conducted and the Startling*

Implications for Diet, Weight Loss, and Long-term Health, Dr. T. Colin Campbell examines the connection between nutrition and heart disease. In fact, the *New York Times* recognized the <u>study</u> as the "Grand Prix of epidemiology" and the "most comprehensive large study ever undertaken of the relationship between diet and the risk of developing disease." If you are only going to read one book, this is my number-one recommendation.

Let's take a look at Jim Fixx, who wrote the *Complete Book of Running.* He ate meat, and while out running one day, <u>dropped dead</u> at the age of 52 from a heart attack. Fixx was genetically predisposed to heart disease. With a plant-based diet, he might have been able to prevent the issues that killed him.

Breast, brain, bladder, and dozens of other cancers are correlated with an increased consumption of animal products.

You'll note similarities between the B+ Diet and *Eat to Live, How Not to Die,* or *Forks Over Knives.* We are all advocating eating an abundance of fresh raw vegetables, fruits, beans, and whole grains *without* oil. We don't count calories or put limits on raw and cooked vegetables. It's a way of life which results in weight loss.

The media has fallen in love with the Mediterranean Diet. It generally encourages fresh produce, beans and legumes, whole grains, and nuts and seeds. However, there is a myth perpetuated that olive oil is good for us, and I disagree! All oils, including olive oil, contain a whopping 14 grams of fat per tablespoon! Further, an abundance of bread, cheese, and pasta (simple carbohydrates) don't serve your weight-loss options well.

Instead, I recommend using water or veggie broth instead of oil for sautéing, rarely eating pasta, incorporating beans, and choosing whole-grain bread (if consuming it).

Plant-Based and the Environment

Raising livestock takes a hefty toll on the environment. One of the biggest contributors of greenhouse gases are cattle, responsible for a whopping 65% of the livestock sector's emissions. Further, 18% of all land in the United States is devoted to pastures to raise livestock. In turn, those pastures encroach upon habitats for other animals.

In addition to the land needed for the animals themselves, there's also the vast amount of land needed to produce crops to feed the animals. Forks Over Knives reports that the majority of cropland in the United States is not used to produce food that people will eat but to produce crops that animals will eat! Between 2000 and 2010, 80% of the plant proteins produced in the United States were allocated to animal feed.

Milking Your Diet

Humans are the only species that continues to drink milk into adulthood, including milk from other animals. When you were an infant, your body produced an enzyme called lactase which allowed you to break down milk. Most adults no longer produce that enzyme, which is why as much as 75% of the world's adult population is lactose intolerant, suffering some degree of symptoms such as nausea, vomiting, and diarrhea.

Today, the data on dairy is decidedly mixed, with many scientists, including physicians, arguing that the most prudent approach to better health is giving up all dairy. Despite it appearing to help with calcium, milk doesn't help with bone health. A study published in the journal *Pediatrics* showed that drinking milk does not improve bone strength in children. More significant in terms of our conversation is the relationship between high fat in milk and cheese and the cancer-causing concerns. Diets high in fat, and especially in saturated fat, can increase the risk of heart disease and stroke and can cause other serious health problems. Some studies show that consumption of dairy products has been linked to higher risk for various cancers, especially to cancers of the reproductive system.

RESOURCES

Books

What the Health: The Startling Truth Behind the Foods We Eat, by Kip Andersen and Keegan Kuhn (2018)

The China Study: The Most Comprehensive Study of Nutrition Ever Conducted, by T. Colin Campbell and Thomas M. Campbell (2016 revised edition)

The End of the Line: How Overfishing Is Changing the World and What We Eat, by Charles Clover (2006)

Younger Next Year: Live Strong, Fit, and Sexy—Until You're 80 and

Beyond, by Chris Crowley and Henry S. Lodge (2007)

Proteinaholic: How Our Obsession with Meat Is Killing Us and What We Can Do About It, by Garth Davis and Howard Jacobson (2016)

Eat to Live: The Amazing Nutrient-Rich Program for Fast and Sustained Weight Loss, by Joel Fuhrman (2011 revised edition)

Whitewash: The Story of a Weed Killer, Cancer, and the Corruption of Science, by Carey Gillam (2017)

How Not to Die: Discover the Foods Scientifically Proven to Prevent and Reverse Disease, by Michael Greger and Gene Stone (2015)

How Not to Diet: The Groundbreaking Science of Healthy, Permanent Weight Loss, by Michael Greger (2019)

Fat Chance: Beating the Odds Against Sugar, Processed Food, Obesity, and Disease, by Robert Lustig (2013)

Fit from Within: 101 Simple Secrets to Change Your Body and Your Life - Starting Today and Lasting Forever by Victoria Moran, (2003)

Main Street Vegan: Everything You Need to Know to Eat Healthfully and Live Compassionately in the Real World by Victoria Moran, (2013)

The Love-Powered Diet: Eating for Freedom, Health, and Joy by Victoria Moran, (2009)

Salt Sugar Fat: How the Food Giants Hooked Us, by Michael Moss (2014)

Beyond Beef: The Rise and Fall of the Cattle Culture, by Jeremy Rifkin (1993)

The Food Revolution: How Your Diet Can Help Save Your Life and Our World, by John Robbins (2010)

Diet for a New America: How Your Food Choices Affect Your Health, Happiness and the Future of Life on Earth, by John Robbins (2012 edition)

Finding Ultra: Rejecting Middle Age, Becoming One of the World's Fittest Men, and Discovering Myself, by Rich Roll (2013 revised edition)

Forks Over Knives: The Plant-Based Way to Health, edited by Gene Stone (2011)

Documentaries

Blackfish (2013)
Cowspiracy (2014)
Diet Fiction (2019)
Earthlings (2005)
Eating You Alive (2018)
Fat, Sick and Nearly Dead (2010)
Food Matters (2008)
Food, Inc. (2008)
Forks Over Knives (2011)
Hungry for Change (2012)
May I Be Frank (2010)
PlantPure Nation (2011)
The Big Fat Lie (2018)
The Game Changers (2018)
Vegucated (2011)
What the Health (2017)

IN A NUTSHELL

1. Eliminating animal products from your diet by default forces you to focus on vegetables, beans, legumes, and whole grains, which improve your health and your weight loss.
2. If you can only make one change toward a vegan diet, my recommendation is to give up dairy. Giving up high-fat cheese and milk reduces your risk of heart disease and cancer.
3. Do your research. Please take the time to consider watching one of the many documentaries free on the streaming services on the benefits of eliminating or reducing your dependence on animal products; it will help your health and the environment.

CHAPTER 20

The Sweet and the Sour

Why Hitting Goal Weight Is Hard and Maintaining Is Even Harder

"Accomplishment will prove to be a journey, not a destination." —Dwight D. Eisenhower

Why Losing Is Winning Only Half the Battle

You are a hero! You achieved your goal. Wow! You're done, right? Wrong!

A staggering 90% of people who lose weight will gain it all back, and often more than they lost (I did every time). In fact, I'd wager everyone who is reading this book today has successfully lost weight. Look at it this way: approximately five million diet books are sold every year, yet I can't find a figure for the number of weight-loss maintenance books sold every year.

Heck, if you remember from chapter 1, I am the Queen of the Weight Lost-and-Found Department: I lost weight on every single diet plan and gained every ounce back. Why? Because I saw my goal weight as a finish line, reinforcing the diet mental-ity of being "on" and "off" a diet.

Bite-Sized Nugget

It's delusional to think you can eat how you used to eat and still look the way you want to look. Your metabolism hasn't changed!

Today, we are on a lifelong journey which never ends. All of the good habits which got us to the point where we are (at our healthy weight) need to be maintained and reinforced. Maintenance is our number-one goal. For the rest of our life, we will be:

1. Eating veggies
2. Having a protein at every meal
3. Drinking tons of water
4. Tracking our food
5. Weighing ourselves daily

The changes you make daily need to be closely monitored and analyzed. You can add in more flavor enhancers checking how your body and weight responds. For example, if I choose to have something different than what I would normally choose and my weight goes up the next day, I pay attention. The lesson: immediately go back to my core plan limiting those foods.

Don't forget our mantra of "out of sight = out of mind." If your downfall was bread, please don't bring it into the house! If you demolish ice cream and call a pint a single serving, commit to only indulging outside of your house. These are the old habits which got us to an unhappy weight and kept us there.

Establish a Maintenance Goal Range

Maintenance will be your lifelong balance of tinkering with what works and what doesn't to keep your weight within a healthy range. Weighing yourself daily will immediately show you the results of your choices. If you keep adding flavor enhancers, for example, without weighing yourself daily, you're back to operating in a vacuum without good data! Now, when you see the scale inching up, you can nip it in the bud and take corrective action. I recommend a maintenance goal range of 5 pounds. For example, my weight range is 123–128 pounds.

It's Harder to Maintain than Lose

I'll be the first to shock you by stating that it's actually harder to maintain your goal weight than to lose the weight. Research suggests that our metabolism acts like a spring that wants to reset your weight to what it was, and other factors play a role too.

Do you remember getting accolades for losing weight? Remember your friends gushing with envy over your weight loss? Those days are now over. You now look the way you want to always look. For the first time, people will meet you and see you as a healthy person, not an overweight person. And that is a good thing! But it also means you have lost the power of positive reinforcement to remain on the weight-loss track.

Bite-Sized Nugget

Find and celebrate non-scale victories to provide the positive reinforcement you won't be getting from friends and family.

Introducing Non-scale Victories

Since we are committed to living our lives at our current goal weight, we must celebrate victories apart from the scale. Put another way: your weight-loss journey created a celebration every time you lost a pound or two. Now, we must substitute joy and gratitude for things that don't show up on our weight scale.

Here are examples of my non-scale victories:

1. Knowing that every single day, when I walk in, everything in my closet fits.

3. I no longer need and will never need an airplane seat belt extender.
4. I never have to worry about a chair collapsing under my weight.
5. I don't have to use the disabled restroom because I couldn't maneuver in a regular-sized stall.
6. I can cross my legs and easily tuck my legs under me.
7. I don't have to ask for a table instead of a booth because I can't fit into a booth. (Yep, I've been stuck in a booth!)
8. I can hop on any amusement park ride knowing that I'll fit and not exceed the weight limit.
9. I can zip-line down a Costa Rican rain forest! (I wasn't able to do this activity when I was there, as the harness would not fit around my waist.)
10. I can hike up to the top of Arthur's Seat—the highest point in Edinburgh, Scotland. (I couldn't kiss the blarney stone in Ireland as I couldn't climb the stairs.)
11. I can jump in a pool and go swimming without embarrassment.
12. I can invest in an expensive coat knowing it will fit today and tomorrow and always.

Don't forget the health and wellness celebrations of your weight loss. Are you off any medications? Did you lower your cholesterol? Can you easily hike a flight of stairs? Are you jogging with a friend? Are you no longer at risk for type 2 diabetes? If any of these questions cause you to answer with a resounding "Yes," then you get to celebrate!

Do you see how I created my list of non-scale victories? You can too. I would love to see your list! Keep comparing now to then to stay motivated. If necessary, turn your non-scale victories upside down. For example, if I revert to my old ways, I won't be able to fit into my clothes. If I revert to my old ways, I might break a chair.

Let's Talk Body Image

Lately, there's tons of media coverage about positive body image. Lizzo champions her size, as does plus-size model Ashley Graham. Yet here we are on different paths. I believe there's a difference between loving yourself and accepting yourself at every weight and giving up and telling yourself you'll always be obese, as in Lizzo's case. If you are reading this book, you are determined and have made the decision to change your life.

Don't get me wrong: Self-love is important. You must live your life every day regardless of your weight and who is watching. Don't deny yourself a beach day because you hate how you look in a bathing suit. If you're on this program, you are on the right path, and your bathing suit will change. Soon, none of your old clothes will fit you.

I get asked this question by my clients at least twice per week: Have I had my excess skin removed? The answer is no.

There remains under my skin a woman who used to weigh 350+ pounds; in some ways, she is still there. But I'm loving me. I lost the weight, and I'm committed to staying at my goal weight.

Find a Coach—Now!

When I look back at what took me to success, it was that I cut through the denial and the excuses. I had a coach and I coached others. I could not turn my back on my clients and lie to them. I was held accountable. Becoming a coach was my first step to accepting accountability.

If you're serious about losing the weight, join me. I have Facebook groups, small groups, and private one-on-one coaching to support your goals. I will tell you that as a coach:

1. **I am honest.** If you want to hear your own rhetoric, you don't need me.
2. **I am judgment free.** No matter what you've chosen to eat, I'm sure I've eaten more. (Remember the number of onion rings I ordered?)
3. **I have empathy.** I clearly have been where you are and can guide you to your promised land of weight-loss goal.
4. **I will give you honest advice.** I guarantee you that you will hit a plateau at some point and lose motivation. I'll review your plan and see where you might have gone off course.

5. **I will hold you accountable.** It's easy to give up on our-selves, but not when we are held accountable by others. I'll stay with you on the journey. I always know that "no news is bad news." Whenever someone disappears from my groups, it's not because they've magically hit goal weight. It's because they went off the plan.

6. **I will bust through your excuses.** You are not a food addict, you probably don't have a thyroid issue, and I don't care if your husband, son, wife, or mother won't support you on this plan. I will. There is always a way to make this program work.

I am here for you. Connect with me for how I can support you on your journey.

Judi@JudiFinneran.com
Facebook: https://www.facebook.com/JudiAFinneran
Website: https://thebplusdiet.com/
Instagram: https://www.instagram.com/judifinneran/
2B Mindset: https://tinyurl.com/2bveganmindset

FREE BONUS MATERIAL

Register Your Book Today and Get Valuable Bonus Material to Lose the Weight and Keep it Off!

I get it: losing weight is hard and keeping it off is even harder. I've assembled a host of goodies to help you with preparing, shopping, and tracking your food and goals. Just sign up here: www.TheBPlusDiet.com/bonus

Here's what you get for free just by signing up in one quick click:

1. **Food Tracker** – One of my core principles is "if you bite it, you write it." Folks who tracked every single bite lost twice as much weight as those who didn't.

2. **Gadget List** – After years of following my program, I've assembled a list of simple gadgets that help you in food prep. Nab it now!

3. **Weight Log** – You must weigh yourself daily. This easy log lets you see your progress in action.

4. **100 Day Tennis Shoe Tracker** – Since I believe in visual reminders and accomplishments of goals, I'vecreated a 100-day tracker. Set a goal and then color in every time you achieve that goal. Whether it's exercis-ing daily, drinking your water, or avoiding alcohol, this is your way to see progress and results.

5. **Meal Planner** – Since planning your meal is the secret recipe for success, I recommend creating your meals one week at a time. This handy planner let's you see at a glance what you'll be eating, take notes and even keep a grocery list.

To your success, Judi